Semantic Processing
Theory and Practice

Semantic Processing

Theory and Practice

Edited by

WENDY BEST PhD,
Birkbeck College,
KAREN BRYAN PhD AND JANE MAXIM PhD
University College London

W
WHURR PUBLISHERS
LONDON AND PHILADELPHIA

© 2000 Whurr Publishers
First published 2000 by
Whurr Publishers Ltd
19b Compton Terrace, London N1 2UN, England and
325 Chestnut Street, Philadelphia PA 19106, USA

Reprinted 2001

British Library Cataloguing in Publication Data
A catalogue record for this book is available from the
British Library.

ISBN: 1 86156 185 7

Printed and bound in the UK by Athenaeum Press Ltd,
Gateshead, Tyne & Wear

Contents

v

Contributors

Wendy Best
Birkbeck College,
University of London

Maria Black
University College London

Karen Bryan
University College, London

Shula Chiat
City University, London

Alison Constable
University College London

Elaine Funnell
Royal Holloway, University of
London

Helen Griffiths
Manchester Royal Infirmary,
Manchester

Susan Kemper
University of Kansas

Joseph P. Levy
University of Greenwich, London

Jane Maxim
University College London

Lyndsey Nickels
Macquarie University, Sydney

Laureen O'Hanlon
University of Kansas

Julie S. Snowden
Manchester Royal Infirmary,
Manchester

Rosemary Varley
University of Sheffield

Kim Zabihi
University College London

Preface

Is it the case that our concepts for fruit are organised and processed differently from those for vehicles? Are the meaning systems for different categories tied closely to the senses through which items are perceived or are they represented separately from sensory systems in pure and abstract form, with different categories represented in similar ways? Are thought processes dependent on the language we have available to express them? How are abstract ideas understood? The ways in which we process meaning are central to our understanding of the world. This book does not provide clear answers to these questions but illustrates a number of different approaches and viewpoints from which the reader can select according to their interests.

The book brings together different ways of looking at how our meaning systems might be structured. The chapters we selected span investigations from different disciplines including psychology, linguistics and speech and language therapy. They include views on semantic processing based on work with children, older adults and with those with impaired meaning systems and on treatment for such disorders.

The book is aimed at a wide audience, from undergraduate psychologists and linguists to practising clinicians working with children or adults with impaired semantic processing.

In 1997 when planning began, we hoped to write the book so that it could be published in the first year of the new century. We achieved our aim but it was at the cost of an estimated year's worth of Saturdays between us! We are therefore very grateful to friends and family for supporting us through many chapter drafts and to the authors of other chapters for meeting deadlines for drafts and revisions.

Particular thanks go to Ruth Herbert, Julie Hickin and Lyndsey Nickels for helpful comments on the chapter on category-specific semantic disorders, to Jane Marshall, Matt Lambon Ralph and co-editors for comments and many suggestions for change to the penultimate chapter, which supports the existence of two-semantic sub-systems. Also thanks to Susan Clifford and Hitomi Sato whose work with us gave rise to some of the issues discussed in the chapter on Alzheimerís disease. Finally, thanks to Brian Best and Sue Peppe for spotting the devil in the detail of references left out, tautologies and words used in ways inappropriate to their meanings.

Wendy Best, Karen Bryan and Jane Maxim
London October 2000

CHAPTER 1

Models of Semantic Memory

ELAINE FUNNELL

Introduction

This chapter has the straightforward purpose of introducing the reader to a variety of influential models of semantic memory and briefly discussing the strengths and weakness of each, in order to provide a theoretical framework within which to consider the more specific issues discussed in following chapters.

It is helpful to adopt the distinction between semantic memory and episodic memory put forward by Tulving (1972). He proposes that the role of semantic memory is to store the general knowledge that people share – for example, that bananas are long and yellow. This knowledge, semantic memory, is stored separately and stands free from episodic memory – memories of the original context, or contexts, within which individuals have personally acquired such knowledge – for example, the different occasions on which they have eaten a banana.

The aspect of semantic memory with which this chapter is concerned is the semantic knowledge required for the identification of objects and object names. The theories to be discussed give a representative sample of the different approaches taken to the semantic representation of objects and object names.

Section 1 introduces network- and feature-based models involved in the identification of features and category membership, and which are based mainly on sentence verification tasks with normal subjects. Thereafter, the models selected have arisen mainly, but not exclusively, to provide accounts for dissociations of performance observed in neuropsychological subjects. Section 2 describes models which specifically reflect the relationship between word meaning and perception, while Section 3 moves on to theories which propose that semantic memory is composed of systems

1

specialized for processing information in different perceptual domains. These contrast with the theories discussed in Section 4, which argue for an amodal representation for semantic information accessible from all sensory modalities. Finally, Section 5 introduces two computational theories of the representation of particular types of semantic properties.

1. Network and feature comparison models

Network models

Collins and Quillian's (1969) model of the structure of semantic memory was developed from a computer-based memory system developed by Quillian (1968). The model is reproduced in Figure 1 and is intended to be a reference system for storing the identity of a concept in the form of what something is (e.g. a robin is a bird) and the properties that something has (e.g. a robin has a red breast; a robin has wings). Information is stored at nodes organized into levels of knowledge from the most abstract to the most specific. For example, the node for animal is connected with the node for bird, which is connected in turn to the node for robin. Properties are stored at the most relevant level. So, for example, properties that are true of most birds, such as 'has feathers', 'can fly', are stored at the 'animal' level. Properties true of more specific concepts, such as 'has a red breast', are stored with the example, such as 'robin'. Although the structure of the model is hierarchical, information can 'enter' the network at any level. For example, if the task was to decide whether 'A robin is a bird', the words 'robin' and 'bird' would access in parallel the nodes for robin and bird in the network.

Experiments used to test network models have generally asked subjects to verify statements that link concepts together. For example, typical statements might be 'Is a robin a bird?' or 'Is a robin an animal?' The time taken to respond is then measured. The model predicts that statements that connect information from levels that are close together in the network should be responded to more quickly than those that connect information stored at levels that are further apart (Collins and Quillian, 1969). This was shown to be true for correct statements: for example, subjects were faster to decide that a robin is a bird than that a robin is an animal.

Similar predictions can be made for decisions about properties. Properties stored with the concept in questions such as 'Does a robin have a red breast?' would be expected to be answered more quickly than questions about properties stored at a more general level such as 'Can a robin fly?' Again, experiments confirmed these predictions when correct statements were used (Collins and Quillian, 1969).

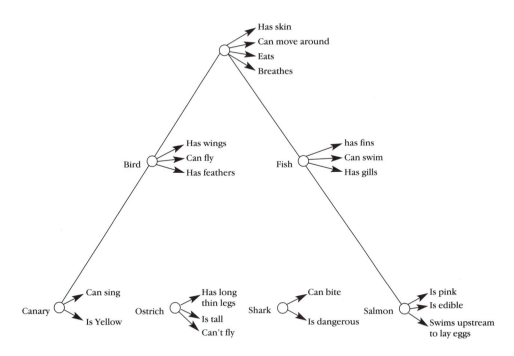

From Collins AM, Quillian MR (1969) Retrieval time from semantic memory. Journal of Verbal Learning and Verbal Behaviour 8: 240–47. Reprinted by permission of Academic Press.

Figure 1. Network model.

However, when negative statements were used, response times failed to support the predictions of the model (Collins and Quillian, 1969; Schaeffer and Wallace, 1970). Subjects were slower to reject statements linking properties stored closer together in the network, such as 'An ostrich can fly', than they were to reject statements linking information stored further apart, such as 'An ostrich has gills'. Schaeffer and Wallace argued that the semantic decisions involved in accepting or rejecting a statement reflect the time involved in making comparisons rather than the structured proximity of information in semantic memory. They argued that the time to make a comparison was affected by the number of features in common between the two items linked together in the statement. Common features helped judgements about correct statements but interfered with incorrect statements, making them harder to reject.

The Collins and Quillian network model was also criticized for its failure to account for the effect of typicality of items in a category (Smith, Shoben and Rips, 1974). Typical members of a category share many properties with other members: for example, an apple is a typical fruit, with characteristics such as roundness, firmness, and juiciness which are shared by many other fruits. In contrast, an atypical member of a category shares few properties with members of the category: for example, a tomato is an atypical fruit. Smith et al. (1974) showed that subjects were faster to decide whether typical members, for example 'robin', belong to the category 'bird', compared with atypical members, such as 'chicken'. More significantly, the opposite was true when subjects were to decide whether typical and atypical birds belonged to the general category of animals. Now, subjects decided that chickens were animals more quickly than they decided that robins were animals. Smith et al. pointed out that these differences in the speed of judgements depending upon the typicality of an item suggested degrees of truth about category membership that were not readily accounted for within the Collins and Quillian model.

Feature models of semantic memory

Lakoff (1972, cited in Smith et al., 1974) noted that statements about category membership vary in truth. Some statements, such as 'A robin is a bird' seemed to be undeniably true; others, such as 'A chicken is a bird' seemed 'technically speaking' to be true; while yet others, such as 'A bat is a bird' seemed 'loosely speaking' to be true. These differences in degree of truth seem to depend upon the extent to which an object can be said to possess the defining features of a category (e.g. a beak, wings, feathers, two legs) and the characteristic features of the individual. Thus, robins and chickens are both unquestionably birds, since they both possess the defining features, but robins share the characteristics of many similar birds, while chickens possess features shared by few other birds. Bats possess some characteristic features of birds, but lack the set that defines the category. Decision times about category membership seem to reflect these differences in truth value: decisions to accept an item as a member of a category are affected positively by the defining features present, but hindered if the characteristic features are relatively uncommon. Decisions to reject the item as a member of the category are speeded if the defining feature set is absent, but slowed if the item has characteristics shared by the category.

Feature models of semantic memory were put forward to explain these differences in truth value and typicality (Schaeffer and Wallace, 1970; Smith et al., 1974). A two-stage feature comparison model was proposed for making decisions about the category membership of an object (Smith et al., 1974). In the first stage, the defining and characteristic features of the object and the defining features of the category are retrieved and compared. If the overlap reaches the criteria set for a good fit, the object is accepted as a member of the category. 'Robin' would be expected to be accepted readily as a member of the category 'bird' at this stage, since it possesses both the defining and characteristic features typical of most birds. If the overlap is so poor that even the lowest acceptable level for a fit fails to be reached then the object is rejected as a member of the category. Those objects, such as 'chicken' and 'bat', that produce an overlap in the shady area between a very good fit and a very poor fit are then subject to the second processing stage, in which only the defining properties of an object are considered. If there is sufficient overlap with the defining features of the category, as in the case of 'chicken', then the object is accepted as a member of the category. If there are insufficient defining features in common, as in the case of 'bat', then the object is rejected as a member of the category.

Spreading activation model of semantic memory

Collins and Loftus (1975) developed the Collins and Quillian (1969) model of semantic structure to account for the evidence that category members vary in typicality. The new model, which is illustrated in Figure 2, consisted of a semantic network of concept nodes organized in terms of semantic similarity. The more properties the concepts share, the more links there are between the two nodes and the closer they are together in the network. When a concept is activated, the activation spreads out along the links of the network to neighbouring concepts. Activation is greatest in links that have been activated often in the past. When presented with a statement such as 'Is a robin a bird?' the nodes for robin and bird are activated as are the links connected to each. If the pathways of links activated by the two concept nodes intersect, then the activation summates and reaches threshold. At this point, the two pathways are then evaluated for semantic relatedness. Words are represented in a separate network that is closely interconnected with the conceptual network.

The notion of spreading activation and the idea of different connection strengths between concepts are strong points in favour of this model. Spreading activation nicely captures the effects of semantic priming demonstrated in normal subjects (Meyer and Schvaneveldt, 1971) and following brain damage (Chertkow, Bub and Seidenberg, 1989); and differences in connection strength are a central feature of current connectionist network models. However, network models in general have been criticized for their lack of constraint. Johnson-Laird, Herrmann and Chaffin (1984) have argued that what one network theory is unable to explain, another (with a slight modification) can explain, making network theories as a class too powerful to be refuted by empirical evidence.

Johnson-Laird et al. (1984) also criticized network models for representing sense relationships rather than reference. They argued that

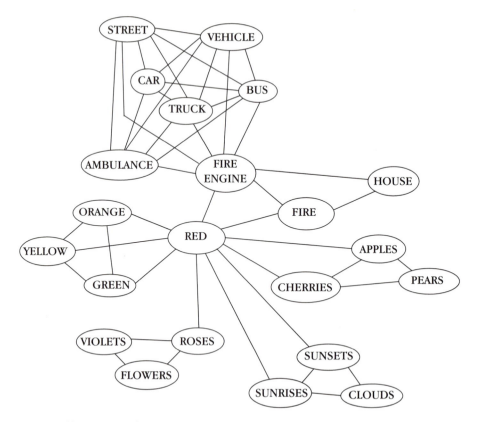

From Collins AM, Loftus MR (1975) A spreading activation theory of semantic processing. Psychological Review 82: 407–28. Copyright © 1975 by the American Psychological Association. Reprinted by permission of the publisher.

Figure 2. Spreading activation model.

cherries and pears are closely linked together because of their common property 'fruit', but the referential, real-world, properties of 'pear' are not represented in the network. Moreover, they suggested that the explicit representation of sense relations may be redundant in the model since knowledge of sense relations may be entailed within the concepts themselves. They argued that if one knows what it is for something to be a pear, and one knows what it is for something to be a fruit, then one knows that a pear is a fruit; thus, this information does not need to be represented explicitly in the model.

Johnson-Laird et al. (1984) pointed out that semantic representations are founded on the fact that human beings can relate language to models of the world. The meanings of words can be properly connected to each other only if they are properly connected to the world. They argued that people construct models of the world on the basis of perception, memory and imagination and that network models failed to capture these dynamic aspects of word meaning.

2. Models of the real world

Paivio's dual coding theory

The relationship between real-world knowledge and words has been addressed directly in some models of semantic processing. Paivio (1978) distinguishes between perceptual and verbal codes in his dual coding theory of semantic memory. In this model, illustrated in Figure 3, perceptual representations (referred to as imagens) are involved in the processing of perceptual images (such as scenes), as well as in generating images and with expressing visual information in drawings. Imagens are linked with verbal representations (referred to as logogens) such that names evoke imagens and imagens evoke names. The verbal system does not contain the perceptible or semantic information that relates to the world, but does contain abstract word logogens that have little reference to the image system. Within each system, representations are associated with other representations: for example, the perceptible representations of dog and cat are linked together, as are their verbal forms in the verbal system.

Processing in this model proceeds over three stages: first comes the level of sensory representation, where incoming sensory information about objects and spoken or written names is registered. Then comes the representational level, where the incoming stimulus activates a symbolic representation of its form: an imagen or a logogen. Next comes the referential level, where connections between the image system and the verbal system allow an image to be named, and a name to arouse an image. Finally comes the associative level where associations between words and associations between images are activated, giving rise to perceptual categorical knowledge related to superordinate names.

Evidence in support of the model bears particularly upon two predictions: first, that memory for information processed by *both* the verbal and non-verbal domains will be superior to information processed by either the verbal or the non-verbal domain; second, that the model predicts interference between processes involved in perception and imagery (Paivio, 1986). Both predictions receive some support from the evidence available. The frequent finding that concrete words with representations in both systems are remembered better than abstract words supports the

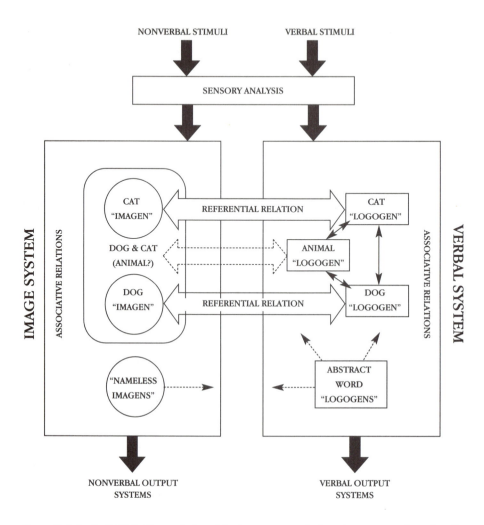

From Paivio A (1978) The relationship between verbal and perceptual codes. In Carterette EC, Friedman MP, (Eds) Handbook of Perception, Vol. 8: Perceptual Coding. London: Academic Press. pp 375–97. Reprinted by permission of the publisher.

Figure 3. Dual coding theory.

first prediction. Experiments such as those which showed interference between the perception of letters representing 'yes' and 'no' responses and the visual imagery of letters (Brooks, 1968) support the second prediction. The strongest claim of the model is the distinction between perceptual and verbal processing. This receives broad support from dissociations between tasks such as object recognition and verbal processing following damage to certain areas of the right and left cerebral hemispheres respectively. However, the model predicts clear dissociations between the processing of pictorial and verbal material following damage to one coding system or the other. As we shall see, such evidence is quite difficult to find.

Allport's model of sensory attribute domains

Allport (1985) also emphasizes the sensory representations of object concepts in semantic memory, but here the sensory representation is shared out – or distributed – across all the sensory attribute domains involved in the processing of the properties of objects. Thus, a concept of a telephone would consist of an amalgamation of the sensory knowledge about its shape, surface texture, sound, size, the actions associated with it, and speech – all represented in different sensory attribute domains. This theory is illustrated in Figure 4. The amalgamation of information occurs because the information in each attribute domain is associated with the information in every other attribute domain, forming an 'auto-associated' pattern of attributes. By activating one sensory attribute of an object

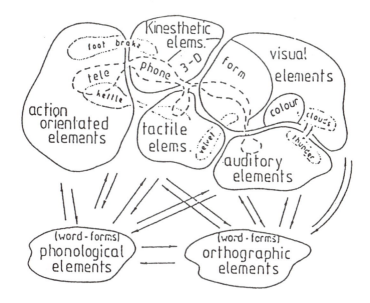

From Allport DA (1985) Distributed memory, modular subsystems and dysphasia. In Newman SK, Epstein R, (Eds) Current Perspectives in Dysphasia. Edinburgh: Churchill Livingstone. pp 32–60. Reprinted by permission of the publisher.

Figure 4. Sensory attribute domains.

concept all the other attributes are activated too. Thus, the sound of a telephone would be linked to information about a telephone's shape, surface pattern, size, and so on. The object concept is represented by the full pattern of auto-associated activation.

Object concepts are represented in the patterns of co-occurring attributes that are established when objects are experienced in the world. In turn, these object concepts act as active pattern recognizers for the future processing of sets of co-occurring properties appearing in the world. As we shall see, the notion that the perceptual properties of objects are both memory representations and active pattern recognizers is included in further models of semantic memory to be discussed later (Riddoch, Humphreys, Coltheart et al., 1988; Coltheart, Inglis, Cupples et al., 1998).

A great strength of Allport's distributed processing model of object concepts is its capacity to predict its behaviour following brain damage. Three predictions are made by Allport (1985) about the effect of brain damage on object concepts. First, since object concepts are represented across a wide variety of attributes, they will be vulnerable only to widespread or diffuse brain damage. Second, object concepts represented by fewer attribute domains (for example, clouds or colours) will be more vulnerable to damage than those represented by a wider variety of attribute domains. Third, loss of particular attribute information should be accompanied by a perceptual deficit for the same information; for example, a loss of perceptual knowledge about what objects look like should be accompanied by a visual agnosia for objects.

The first prediction of the model is well supported by the demonstration that semantic deficits are particularly likely to be found in dementing disorders in which diffuse brain damage is the norm (Hodges and Patterson, 1997). In addition, concepts for objects with fewer attribute domains have been reported to be more affected by brain damage (Nickels and Howard 1995), thus supporting the second prediction of the model. The third prediction of an association between a loss of attribute information and a perceptual deficit has received little attention. However, a recent case report (Coltheart et al., 1998) of an individual with a loss of knowledge for particular perceptual attributes (such as 'has legs') provides preliminary support for this prediction. In this case, the perceptual knowledge deficit was accompanied by a perceptual deficit for the processing of perceptual properties of objects presented in pictures.

3. Modality-specific models of semantic memory

While Allport's model integrates information from different sensory modalities into a single – though widely spread – distributed attribute system, some other models do the reverse and break down semantic memory into distinct, or partially distinct, modality-specific conceptual systems. Like Paivio (1978), Warrington (1975) proposed that visual and verbal semantic information might be represented in separable systems. The proposal was initially based on the fact that two subjects with a semantic disorder responded differently to words and pictures: one subject performing better with pictures; the other better with words. Shallice (1987, 1988) based his support for this theory on three different neuropsychological phenomena: a) the modality-specific aphasias; b) modality-specific priming effects; and c) modality-specific aspects of semantic disorders. These three sources of evidence are considered in turn.

First, the modality-specific aphasias: these refer to people who are able to name objects presented in one sensory modality, such as touch, but are unable to name objects presented in another sensory modality, such as vision. This occurs despite the fact that they can identify the visual object sufficiently well to gesture its use or to mention an associated action (e.g. Lhermitte and Beauvois, 1973). Such disorders are hard to explain if the semantic knowledge that supports the ability to gesture resides in the same system that allows objects presented by touch to be identified and named.

Second, the modality-specific priming experiments: these refer to the case of a man who had difficulty reading aloud words and who was better able to name objects from an auditory description than when the objects were presented visually (Warrington and Shallice, 1979). His ability to read aloud words was improved when he was given an auditory prompt (or prime) – such as *Egypt* – while he was struggling to read a word – such as *pyramid*. In comparison, giving him a picture prompt – for example, a picture of a pyramid – was much less helpful. Shallice (1987) argues that the differential benefits of verbal and visual prompts on this man's oral reading is consistent with the operation of separable verbal and visual/pictorial semantic memory systems.

The third source of evidence – the modality-specific aspects of semantic systems – refers to two sources of evidence. The first is based upon the claim that some brain-damaged people respond differently to semantic questions about objects when given either pictures or names (Warrington, 1975). Thus, they may be able to decide that a picture of an object (visual modality) is an animal, but not be able to make the same decision about the name of the object (verbal modality). The second source of evidence is based upon the claim that some people may respond differently when naming pictures or defining the names of the same objects (Warrington and Shallice, 1984). These people may perform more successfully in one task than another but, more importantly, the knowledge available to them in the two tasks may differ. Thus, they may name some items that they cannot define and define some items that they cannot name. When knowledge is available when tested in one modality of presentation (e.g. the visual modality) but not in another (e.g. the verbal modality), then this is taken as evidence that the tasks draw upon different sources of semantic information and that therefore separable semantic systems are involved.

One difficulty with the modality-specific theory of semantic memory was the lack of information about the content of the different semantic systems involved. Riddoch et al., (1988) tried to work out what the properties of the different modality-specific semantic systems might be from the methods employed in the studies used to support the multiple semantic systems hypothesis (Warrington, 1975; Warrington and Shallice, 1984). Since, in these studies, the same questions were asked of verbal and pictorial material, Riddoch et al. inferred that an underlying assumption of the model was that the visual and verbal semantic systems store identical information, each presumably in a format appropriate to the particular input modality. A processing framework that captured this account was put forward by Riddoch et al. and is reproduced in Figure 5.

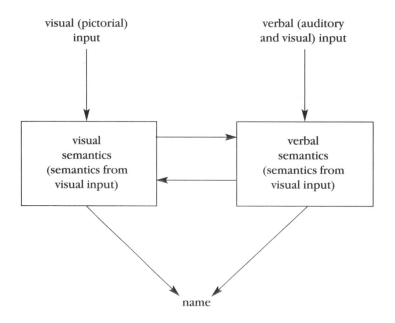

From Riddoch MJ, Humphreys GW, Coltheart M, Funnell E (1988) Semantic system or systems? Neuropsychological evidence re-examined. Cognitive Neuropsychology 5: 3–25. Reprinted by permission of Psychological Press Ltd.

Figure 5. Modality-specific semantic systems.

Subsequently, however, in the most explicit statement to be made about this issue, Shallice (1988) proposed that the visual system contains a variety of information concerning the sensory properties of an object. This included the objects that would be found or used with the object; the appropriate actions to use with the object; its function; any expected behaviour of the object; one's emotional attitude to the object; and its abstract associations. The verbal system would also be expected to contain some of the same information, for example knowledge of function and abstract properties. Because of this shared knowledge, Shallice suggests that the visual and verbal systems must be separable but linked.

4. Amodal models of semantic memory

Overall, the evidence for multiple semantic systems is weak. Riddoch et al. (1988) were able to provide arguments against each of the three sources of evidence for multiple semantic systems proposed by Shallice (1988). In addition, relatively few cases have been reported who provide support for the multiple semantic systems model. In place of a multiple systems account, Riddoch proposed an amodal theory of semantic memory with separate visual and auditory inputs. This is illustrated in Figure 6.

One problem with the multiple semantic systems hypothesis, not discussed so far, has been the application of the term 'modality' to two disparate properties: visual and verbal. While 'visual' implies the modality of presentation, or the visual appearance of a stimulus, 'verbal' implies a connection with language, which might be processed visually and/or aurally. In the model put forward by Riddoch et al., the use of these terms is clarified.

First, the properties of the input materials are divided according to the sensory modality in which they are experienced: visual inputs are pictures and written words; auditory inputs are environmental sounds and spoken words. The visual and verbal inputs are able to access specialized, pre-semantic, perceptual recognition systems. In the visual system these contain the structural descriptions for objects and for written words, and in the auditory system these contain the perceptual descriptions for recognizing environmental sounds and spoken words. These input systems then map on to an amodal semantic system, which contains information about the associations with other concepts and functional characteristics. Bi-directional links between the semantic system and the perceptual systems allow structural descriptions to be expressed in words, and in turn allow words, or thoughts, to activate information about the structural description, for example, in tasks of drawing from memory, or answering questions about object properties. In order to account for optic aphasia (in which an individual is able to gesture the use of a visual object that they are unable to identify) Riddoch et al. argue that the pre-semantic structural description of an object may contain information that can be used to generate actions.

Riddoch et al.'s model has recently been extended by Coltheart et al. (1998) to include multiple perceptual domains (visual, auditory, olfactory and tactile), each with its own perceptual knowledge base about the nature of objects (see Figure 7). This perceptual knowledge is used both as a pattern recognizer for objects in the world and as information in answer to questions about the perceptual properties of named objects. In support of this aspect of the model, Coltheart et al. provide evidence from a single case study to show that when knowledge of perceptual attributes is lost, so too is the ability to process the perceptual attributes of visually presented objects.

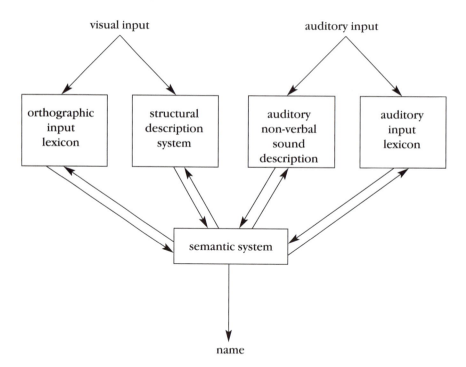

From Riddoch MJ, Humphreys GW, Coltheart M, Funnell E (1988) Semantic system or systems? Neuropsychological evidence re-examined. Cognitive Neuropsychology 5: 3–25. Reprinted by permission of Psychological Press Ltd.

Figure 6. Amodal model of semantic memory.

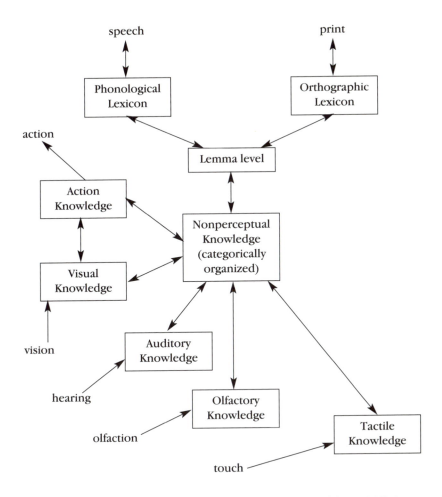

From Coltheart M, Inglis L, Cupples L, Michie P, Bates A, Budd B (1998) A semantic subsystem of visual attributes. Neurocase 4: 353–70. Reprinted by permission of Oxford University Press.

Figure 7. A model of the representation of object knowledge.

In addition to the domain-specific perceptual knowledge bases, the model incorporates a system of action knowledge (that can account for the ability to gesture object use in optic aphasia) and a central non-perceptual semantic knowledge base that is shared by all perceptual domains. An important aspect of this model is that the central semantic knowledge base is organized by semantic category – an important aspect of semantic processing that will be discussed later in this chapter.

The OUCH model

A further amodal model of semantic memory, referred to as the Organized Unitary Content Hypothesis, or OUCH, was put forward by Caramazza, Hillis, Rapp et al. (1990). OUCH differs from the amodal models just discussed (Riddoch et al.,1988; Coltheart et al., 1998) by incorporating perceptual knowledge and action plans within the amodal system itself. The amodal semantic representations in OUCH consist of a network of semantic predicates, such as 'has a handle' or 'has stripes', which are represented in amodal format and which define the meaning of the term. The semantic predicates capture different aspects of meaning, including reference to perceptual features, action patterns, and associations with other objects and concepts. This network of information is accessible to inputs from orthographic and phonological lexical representations of spoken and written words and from structural representations of the perceptual properties of objects. The model is illustrated in Figure 8.

There are two important characteristics of the model. First, information about the structural properties of an object has *privileged access* to the

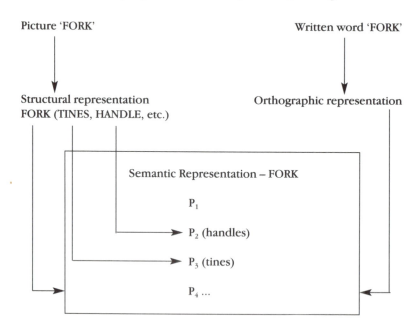

Adapted from Caramazza A, Hillis AE, Rapp BC, Romani C (1990) The multiple semantics hypothesis: multiple confusions? Cognitive Neuropsychology 7: 161–89. Reprinted by permission of Psychological Press Ltd.

Figure 8. The amodal OUCH model of semantic memory.

perceptual predicates of objects. This occurs because perceptual predicates are directly compatible with information received from the structural descriptions. Thus, information from visual structural descriptions has privileged access to semantic predicates that describe visual properties. Likewise, information from tactile structural descriptions has privileged access to semantic predicates that describe tactile properties of objects; and so on for auditory input, taste, etc. Privileged access means that the information pertaining to a particular input modality can be accessed *directly* from the structural descriptions specific to that modality and in parallel to the processes involved in accessing the full set of predicates. Privileged access may apply to whole objects or to object parts. In contrast, names provide only an address to the full network of predicates, none of which has privileged access relative to any others.

The second important characteristic of the model is that of *privileged relationships* within the network itself. That is, the connections between the semantic predicates in the network do not all have equal strength. Particularly strong links are argued to be formed between visual perceptual predicates and the actions that may be performed on them. This occurs because of the strong association between objects and their use in the real world. These associations are thought to be stronger than associations made between other aspects of meaning.

Two predictions are made about the behaviour of the OUCH model following damage to the system. First, strong links between predicates are more likely to be spared than weaker ones. Second, if the connections between the structural descriptions and the semantic network representing a particular object concept are damaged, then the semantic predicates most likely to be accessed successfully are those with privileged links. These properties of the model are argued to explain the modality-specific aphasias. For example, a person with optic aphasia can gesture but not name a visually presented object. This arises when there is a selective deficit for computing the full semantic representation from the visual structural descriptions of a visually presented object. When this occurs, the links giving direct, privileged access to the semantic predicates that represent perceptual attributes continue to operate. Since these perceptual predicates are more strongly linked to actions than to the full set of predicates required for specific names, the subject is able to gesture the use of the object though unable to provide the name. Spared ability to name the object from a verbal description would be based on spared access to the full set of semantic properties from verbal input. In this way the model accounts for the phenomenon of optic aphasia *within* the structure of the semantic system. This contrasts with the alternative proposal that the ability to gesture the use of a visual object which is unable to be named is an emergent property of information activated within the structural descriptions (Riddoch et al., 1988).

An attempt to evaluate the OUCH model was made by Chertkow, Bub and Caplan (1992) who tested three predictions that they argued followed from the model when the semantic properties were damaged. First, picture stimuli should produce better performance than names. Second, picture stimuli should give rise to better performance with perceptual questions (tapping into perceptual predicates) than with associative questions (tapping into the network of semantic predicates). Third, that pictures of objects with many structurally distinct parts (and therefore many privileged perceptual links to semantics) should be better recognized than objects with fewer structurally distinct parts. These predictions were tested with a group of people with probable Alzheimer's disease. The group showed an advantage for processing pictures of objects compared with their spoken names, confirming the first prediction. However, they failed to answer perceptual questions more successfully to pictures than to words or to show better recognition of objects with many distinct parts: thus failing to confirm the second and third predictions of the model.

To explain their data, Chertkow et al. (1992) proposed a separation between associative knowledge, which they suggested is represented in an amodal store, and the semantic information necessary for identifying visually presented objects, which they suggested is composed of both perceptual and functional knowledge. They argued that this information is semantic rather than structural and so distinguished it from the structural descriptions of the Riddoch et al. model which are considered to be purely perceptual. In response to the criticisms of OUCH, Hillis, Rapp and Caramazza (1995) argued that Chertkow et al. had misinterpreted their model; that predictions 2 and 3 did not follow from it; and that the data of Chertkow et al. were, in fact, consistent with the OUCH model. They noted, however, the value of such tests of the model in sharpening the theoretical and empirical methods involved in studying semantic memory.

5. Models of semantic properties/ property-specific models of semantic memory

The arguments in the previous section have concentrated on whether or not there are separable semantic systems for different modalities of processing (e.g. vision and touch) or different types of materials (pictures or words). In the class of model to be described next, the issue of interest moves away from different modalities to different types of semantic properties. Of these, consideration of the distinction between concrete and abstract properties has had the longest history and will be discussed first.

Abstract and concrete semantic properties

In memory tasks, normal subjects generally process concrete words more quickly and accurately than abstract words. Concrete words are also read aloud much more successfully than abstract words in the acquired reading disorder referred to as 'deep dyslexia' (Marshall and Newcombe, 1973; Coltheart, Patterson and Marshall, 1987). In this reading disorder, subjects make errors, such as reading *berry* as 'grapes', and *daughter* as 'sister', in which the response is related to the target in meaning, but neither looks nor sounds like the target word. The similarity in meaning between the target and response has suggested that the word is read aloud by a system which first finds the meaning of the written word and then finds a spoken word form to name the meaning. Semantic errors are thought to occur when the ability to find the precise meaning in semantic memory is disrupted. The fact that concrete words are read so much more success-fully than abstract words by the semantic system, has suggested that the semantic processes concerned with concrete words are at least partially separated from the semantic processes concerned with abstract words (Morton and Patterson, 1980). Occasional case reports of people whose processing shows the reverse effect by producing superior performance on abstract words compared with concrete words (Warrington 1981; Warrington, 1975) have lent support to the view that concrete and abstract words map on to semantic systems with different characteristics.

Plaut and Shallice (1993) have modelled dissociations between concrete and abstract words in oral reading tasks in a distributed connec-tionist model of reading. In this model, the meaning of abstract words is represented mainly by abstract properties, of which there are relatively few, and the meaning of concrete words is represented mainly by concrete properties, of which there are relatively many. The allocation of different numbers of semantic properties to concrete and abstract words was based on work by Jones (1985) which suggested that abstract words are repre-sented by fewer semantic predicates (measured by statements such as 'A dog has four legs', 'An idea is a thought') than are concrete words. In the Plaut and Shallice model there is also very little overlap between the semantic properties accessed by concrete and abstract words in this semantic system.

The architecture of the model is illustrated in Figure 9. The model connects orthographic representations, for recognizing written word forms, with their semantic representations (via a set of hidden units). The semantic representations are connected in turn with a set of phonological representations, representing spoken word forms (via a further set of hidden units). There are no interconnections between properties within the semantic system. However, there is a set of bi-directional connections between semantic units and a set of 'clean-up' units. These connections link together semantic properties that regularly occur together in word meanings, allowing combinations of properties to influence each other directly. The clean-up units play a greater role in connecting together semantic properties of concrete words which are more numerous, than the less numerous properties of abstract words.

When the normally operating system is damaged, by removing some connections or by introducing noise into the system, the processing of concrete words is most upset by damage to the clean-up units. In contrast,

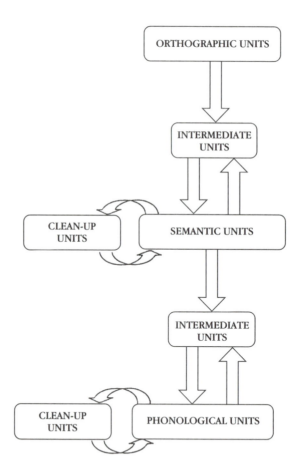

From Plaut D, Shallice T (1993) Deep dyslexia: a case study of connectionist neuro-psychology. Cognitive Neuropsychology 7: 161–90. Reprinted by permission of Psychological Press Ltd.

Figure 9. Connectionist model of the processing of concrete and abstract words.

the processing of abstract words is most upset by damage to the connections between the orthographic and semantic units. Thus, the model can simulate both deep dyslexia (in which concrete words are spared relative to abstract words) and concrete word dyslexia (in which abstract words are spared relative to concrete words).

There are several reasons for doubting the validity of the model as a description of the structure of semantic memory in human subjects. Recent work has shown that although normal subjects generate more properties to concrete words than to abstract words *overall*, the number of features overlap considerably and fail to separate the two classes of words (De Mornay Davies, 1997; De Mornay Davies and Funnell, in press). In addition, the effectiveness of the simulations owes much to the orthographic similarity between pairs of concrete and abstract words (e.g. *tart–tact*; *wave–wage*) on which the model is trained, and can be argued to be unrepresentative of the orthographic similarities found in the vocabulary of human beings (Funnell, 1999).

Particularly pertinent, however, is recent evidence reported by Marshall, Chiat and Pring (1996) suggesting that it may be a mistake to think of abstract properties as generally restricted to abstract words, and concrete properties to concrete words. Rather, it seems that concrete words have meanings that contain both concrete and abstract descriptions. As the result of a stroke, an individual studied by Marshall et al. was found to name abstract words more successfully than concrete words. In addition, his ability to name concrete words in response to a definition was influenced by the concreteness of the context in which the meaning was set. Thus, an abstract description, such as 'A fortified, historic building' was more successful in eliciting the naming response 'castle' than was a concrete description, such as 'A building with turrets and a drawbridge'. His performance suggests that the meanings of concrete words include both concrete and abstract properties. Plaut and Shallice's model, which assigns abstract properties almost completely to abstract words, would not generalize to these findings.

Category specificity and visual and functional properties of objects

Models of semantic memory have been concerned recently with the representation of visual and semantic properties of concrete objects. Arguments for a distinction between representations of visual and functional semantic properties have emerged from the study of category-specific disorders of semantic memory. In these disorders, people have difficulty identifying objects belonging to particular semantic categories, such as animals or artefacts. There is much controversy about the underlying explanations for these category-specific disorders. Studies have been criticized for the lack of control of variables, such as concept familiarity and visual complexity, across categories (Stewart, Parkin and Hunkin,1992; Funnell and Sheridan, 1992). And the greater visual similarity within categories of living things has been argued to be a contributory factor to disorders mostly affecting living things (Gaffan and Heywood, 1993). Arguments have also been made for the need for a principled account of the multitude of different patterns of category-specific disorder reported (Caramazza and Shelton, 1998). Here, we shall introduce one model of an influential theory of semantic processing that was put forward to account for disorders that mainly affected either artefacts or living things.

This category-specific theory was put forward originally by Warrington and Shallice (1984). They noted that some people had been reported with deficits mainly affecting the recognition of artefacts while others had been reported with deficits mainly affecting the recognition of living things, although some exceptions to these broad category distinctions were reported that will not be considered here. To explain the broad distinction between categories, they suggested that artefacts are recognized mainly by their strong functional roles while living things are more dependent upon their visual appearance. If the semantic system represents functional and visual features independently, then damage to functional features would be expected to affect artefacts more than living things, while damage to visual features would be expected to affect living things more than artefacts. Thus, in this theory, category-specific deficits are viewed as an emergent property of damage to underlying visual or functional property systems. This theory has been termed the sensory-functional theory (Caramazza and Shelton, 1998).

To test this theory, Farah and McClelland (1991) collected dictionary definitions for a set of living and non-living things, and found a greater proportion of visual properties compared to functional properties for living things than was found for non-living things. These differing proportions were used to set up the computational model of semantic memory illustrated in Figure 10. In this model, visual and functional features of objects are depicted in separable systems but linked by bi-directional connections. Input systems are separated into a verbal system for written and spoken words, and a pictorial visual input system. Each input system has bi-directional connections to functional and visual semantic units.

The model was trained to produce the correct semantic pattern to 10 living and 10 non-living things. In line with the ratios obtained from dictionary definitions, the living things were represented by an average of 16.1 visual and 2.1 functional units, while nonliving things were represented by an average of 9.4 visual and 6.7 functional units. All semantic patterns contained visual and functional units. When presented with each picture pattern the network was trained to produce the correct semantic pattern and name pattern. Likewise, when presented with each name pattern, the model was trained to produce the correct semantic pattern and picture pattern.

When the model was fully trained to produce the correct responses, damage was inflicted to either the visual or functional semantic units. Semantic representations of living things were most affected by damage to visual semantic units, while semantic representations of non-living things were most affected by damage to functional units. The greater the damage to the system, the more adverse the effects. Marked damage to visual semantic units also affected non-living things, because severe reduction in activation between visual and functional units reduced the 'critical mass' of activated semantic units necessary to activate a name or a picture.

Farah and McClelland note that the ability of the model to simulate category-specific disorders depends upon the fact that there is a relationship between the type of category (living or non-living) and the type of semantic property (visual or functional) on which its semantic representation most depends. They note also several limitations to the model. First, the model is limited to visual and functional information and does not include information about tactile and auditory domains. Second, functional semantics could have been subdivided into more specific

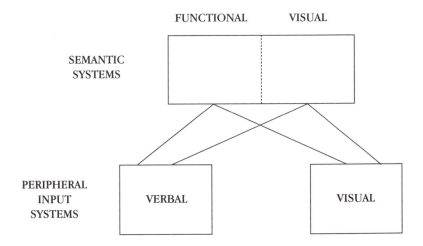

From Farah MJ, McClelland JL (1991) A computational model of semantic memory impairment: modality specificity and emergent category specificity. Journal of Experimental Psychology: General 120: 339–57. Copyright © 1991 by the American Psychological Association. Reprinted by permission of the publisher.

Figure 10. Parallel distributed processing model of 'category-specific' effects.

components. Third, name and picture inputs should vary in the nature of their relation to semantic units. Fourth, the pictorial units should have closer links with visual semantic units than functional links. Finally, the performance of the model is based upon the pattern of activated units and is a different measure to those used to measure human performance.

Caramazza and Shelton (1998) observed that the empirical basis for the different proportions of sensory and functional features used in Farah and McClelland's model depends upon a narrow interpretation of 'functional' to mean 'what an object is used for'. They argue that this biases the size of the count of functional features towards that of artefacts. They showed that when the notion of function was broadened to include information about where an object is found, and other characteristics, such as what it eats and how it behaves, then equivalent ratios of visual to functional features were produced for living and non-living things. This finding is argued to challenge the Farah and McClelland model since its ability to simulate category-specific disorders depends directly upon an imbalance in the assignment of visual and functional properties to the two categories. Clearly, the validity of any particular property-based theory of semantic memory depends upon the criteria used to define the properties. In order to arbitrate between models, empirical data (based upon human perform-ance) are required to determine what comprises the functional properties of objects.

Caramazza and Shelton (1998) also argue that two predictions of the sensory/functional theory of category-specific deficits are not supported by findings in the literature. The first is that subjects should not be found whose performance differs across categories that are strongly represented by visual features, such as animals and fruit/vegetables. They note, however, that cases can be found in the literature where *either* the category of animals *or* the category of fruit/vegetables is impaired. The second predic-tion is that category-specific impairments should be related to proportional differences in knowledge of visual and functional properties: difficulties identifying living things should be associated with more deficits to know-ledge of visual features compared with functional features; conversely, specific difficulties with non-living things should show the reverse effect. They note, however, that there are now a number of reports of cases of difficulty in identifying living things in which both knowledge of visual and knowledge of functional properties appear to be equally impaired.

Caramazza and Shelton (1998) argue that category-specific disorders can be accounted for within the OUCH model (Caramazza et al., 1990) if the semantic properties that are shared by members of a category are stored closely together in semantic space. This argument, however, is reminiscent of the spreading activation model of Collins and Loftus (1975) and entails all the problems associated with network models that were discussed earlier. Brain-damage affecting different regions of semantic space would then give rise to category-specific effects, the nature of which would depend upon which area of semantic space had been affected.

Although satisfied that OUCH can explain the appearance of category-specific disorders, Caramazza and Shelton were puzzled as to why, within a system where brain damage might be expected to affect all categories equally often, a disorder affecting living things happens to be particularly prevalent. As a solution to this problem, they suggested that evolutionary constraints give rise to the development of neural mechanisms specialized for processing domains of knowledge that are particularly significant for survival. These are argued to consist of separate domains of knowledge specialized for the recognition of animals, plants and (perhaps) artefacts. Within this account, category-specific semantic disorders are argued to reflect genuine distinctions between different domains of knowledge – for example, knowledge of animals can be impaired relative to plants – rather than damage to broad domains of knowledge, such as living things and artefacts, or to particular types of property.

Closing comments

This brief introduction to models of semantic memory may well have left the reader with feelings of dissatisfaction and uncertainty. Dissatisfaction, because of the disparate nature of the models, leaving perhaps a feeling of incompatibility and incoherence; uncertainty, because no model seems to be even partially satisfactory as a model of semantic memory that can be applied to all data and all relevant theoretical questions. If so, then these feelings reflect the state of the art at present. The various models illustrate the disjointed development of work in the field. They arise from different theoretical questions; different methods for deriving data; and different sources and patterns of data. Semantic memory is a vast human resource with potentially many different dimensions. It might help the reader if the models discussed here can be viewed as attempts to understand particular aspects of this complex system rather than as attempts to account for the structure of semantic memory as a whole.

References

Allport DA (1985) Distributed memory, modular subsystems and dysphasia. In Newman SK, Epstein R, (Eds) Current Perspectives in Dysphasia. Edinburgh: Churchill Livingstone. pp 32–60.

Brooks LR (1968) Spatial and verbal components of the act of recall. Canadian Journal of Psychology 22: 349–68.

Caramazza A, Hillis AE, Rapp BC, Romani C (1990) The multiple semantics hypothesis: multiple confusions? Cognitive Neuropsychology 7: 161–89.

Caramazza A, Shelton JR (1998) Domain-specific knowledge systems in the brain: the animate-inanimate distinction. Journal of Cognitive Neuroscience 10: 1–34.

Chertkow H, Bub D, Seidenberg M (1989) Priming and semantic memory loss in Alzheimer's disease. Brain and Language 36: 420–46.

Chertkow H, Bub D, Caplan D (1992) Constraining theories of semantic memory processing: evidence from dementia. Cognitive Neuropsychology 9: 327–365.

Collins AM, Loftus MR (1975) A spreading activation theory of semantic processing. Psychological Review 82: 407–28.

Collins AM, Quillian MR (1969) Retrieval time from semantic memory. Journal of Verbal Learning and Verbal Behaviour 8: 240–47.

Coltheart M, Inglis L, Cupples L, Michie P, Bates A, Budd B (1998) A semantic subsystem of visual attributes. Neurocase 4: 353–70.

Coltheart M, Patterson K, Marshall J, (Eds) (1987) Deep Dyslexia. London and New York: Routledge and Kegan Paul.

De Mornay Davies P (1997) The Semantic Representation of Concrete and Abstract Words. Unpublished PhD thesis. Royal Holloway University of London.

De Mornay Davies P, Funnell E (in press). Semantic representation and ease of predication. Brain and Language.

Farah MJ, McClelland JL (1991) A computational model of semantic memory impairment: modality specificity and emergent category specificity. Journal of Experimental Psychology: General 120: 339–57.

Funnell E (1999) Deep dyslexia. In Funnell E, (Ed) Classic Cases in the Neuropsychology of Reading. Hove: Psychology Press.

Funnell E, Sheridan J (1992) Categories of knowledge? Unfamiliar aspects of living and nonliving things. Cognitive Neuropsychology 9: 135–53.

Gaffan D, Heywood CA (1993) A spurious category-specific visual agnosia for living things in normal human and nonhuman primates. Journal of Cognitive Neuroscience 5: 118–28.

Hillis AE, Rapp B, Caramazzo A (1995) Constraining claims about theories of semantic memory – more on unitary versus multiple sematics. Cognitive Neuropsychology 12(2): 175–186.

Hodges JR, Patterson K (1997) Semantic memory disorders. Trends in the Cognitive Neurosciences 1: 68–72.

Johnson-Laird PN, Herrmann DJ, Chaffin R (1984) Only connections: a critique of semantic networks. Psychological Bulletin 96: 292–315.

Jones GV (1985) Deep dyslexia, imageability, and ease of predication. Brain and Language 24: 1–19.

Lakoff G (1972) Hedges: A study in meaning criteria and the logic of fuzzy concepts. In Papers from the eighth Regional meeting of the Chicago Linguistic Society. Cited in Smith ES, Shoben EJ, Rips LJ (1975). Structure and Process in Sematic Memory: A featural model for semantic decisions. Psychological Review, 81: 214–241.

Lhermitte F, Beauvois MF (1973) A visual-speech disconnection syndrome: report of a case with optic-aphasia, agnosic alexia, and colour agnosia. Brain 96: 695–714.

Marshal JC, Newcombe F (1973) Patterns of paralexia. Journal of Psycholinguistic Research 2: 175–99.

Marshall J, Pring T, Chiat S, Robson J (1996) Calling a salad a federation: an investigation of semantic jargon, Part 1 – Nouns. Journal of Neurolinguistics 9: 237–50.

Meyer DE, Schvaneveldt RW (1971) Facilitation in recognising pairs of words: evidence of a dependence between retrieval operations. Journal of Experimental Psychology 90: 227–34.

Morton J, Patterson K (1980) A new attempt at an interpretation, or an attempt at a new interpretation. In Coltheart M, Patterson K, Marshall JC, (Eds) Deep Dyslexia. London and New York: Routledge and Kegan Paul. pp 91–118.

Nickels LA, Howard D (1995) Aphasic naming: what matters? Neuropsychologia 33: 1281–1303.

Paivio A (1978) The relationship between verbal and perceptual codes. In Carterette EC, Friedman MP, (Eds) Handbook of Perception, Vol. 8: Perceptual Coding. London: Academic Press. pp 375–97

Paivio A (1986) Mental Representations: A Dual Coding Approach. Oxford: Oxford University Press.

Plaut D, Shallice T (1993) Deep dyslexia: a case study of connectionist neuropsychology. Cognitive Neuropsychology 7: 161–90.

Quillian MR (1968) Semantic memory. In. Minsky M, (Ed) Semantic Information Processing. Cambridge, MA: MIT Press. pp 375–97.

Riddoch MJ, Humphreys GW, Coltheart M, Funnell E (1988) Semantic system or systems? Neuropsychological evidence re-examined. Cognitive Neuropsychology 5: 3–25.

Schaeffer B, Wallace R (1970) The comparison of word meanings. Journal of Experimental Psychology 86: 144–52.

Shallice T (1987) Impairments of semantic processing: multiple dissociations. In Coltheart M, Sartori G, Job R, (Eds) The Cognitive Neuropsychology of Language. London: Lawrence Erlbaum Associates.

Shallice T (1988) From Neuropsychology to Mental Structure. Cambridge: Cambridge University Press.

Smith EE, Shoben EJ, Rips LJ (1974) Structure and process in semantic memory: a featural model for semantic decisions. Psychological Review 81: 214–41.

Stewart F, Parkin AJ, Hunkin NM (1992) Naming impairments following recovery from herpes simplex encephalitis: category-specific? Quarterly Journal of Experimental Psychology 44A: 261–84.

Tulving E (1972) Episodic and semantic memory. In Tulving E, Donaldson W, (Eds.) The Organization of Memory. New York: Academic Press

Warrington EK (1975) The selective impairment of semantic memory. Quarterly Journal of Experimental Psychology 27: 635–57.

Warrington EK (1981) Concrete word dyslexia. British Journal of Psychology 72: 175–96.

Warrington EK, Shallice T (1979) Semantic access dyslexia, Brain 102: 43–63.

Warrington EK, Shallice T (1984) Category-specific impairments. Brain 107: 829–53.

CHAPTER 2

Connectionist modelling of semantic deficits

JOSEPH P. LEVY

Introduction

In recent years theory building in cognitive psychology has been making increasing use of a particular computational framework that has become known as connectionism (or neural network modelling or parallel distributed processing – PDP). Rather than employing the metaphor of the serial computer and describing behaviour at a symbolic level of description, connectionism uses a 'sub-symbolic' or pattern-processing approach that is inspired by the structure of the brain. Like other methods of computer modelling, connectionism allows theories to be tested by actually implementing them as working systems. It has also added to the general theoretical vocabulary of the field by providing new computational primitives and principles that can be employed in theory building.

There are two particularly compelling reasons why many workers in cognitive neuropsychology have also enthusiastically taken these techniques on board. First, connectionism espouses what has been called 'brain style computation'. This implies that, at the very least, broad characteristics of brain structure are reflected in connectionist models, e.g. parallel processing by many relatively simple units and a degree of distribution in the way that information is represented. Second, once built, a model of a particular cognitive ability can be damaged or 'lesioned' and so possibly simulate a neuropsychological deficit. Connectionist models are particularly attractive in this regard because they usually do not fail catastrophically when damaged and so exhibit a kind of graceful degradation in performance that has been compared to what occurs after some types of brain damage.

There are additional reasons why it might be believed that connectionism can add to our understanding of semantic processing. There are several approaches to semantic representation, particularly feature-based approaches, which are conveniently implemented within a connectionist network. Building a computational model based round some particular assumptions about representation allows us to test the repercussions on a scale that would be impossible to do as a thought experiment. For example, the particular examples that we shall see in this chapter allow the testing of semantic representation schemes to see if they can account for the existence and characteristics of category-specific deficits.

This chapter first introduces some of the more important characteristics of connectionist networks, and then surveys the ways in which lexical and conceptual semantics have been represented in connectionist models. Finally the development of a range of connectionist models of category-specific deficits is reviewed, demonstrating the theoretical value of developing computational models to implement hypotheses about semantic representations.

Why do computational modelling?

For the last twenty or thirty years cognitive psychology has been dominated by the *information processing* paradigm, the idea that the mind performs computational processes on different levels of representation. We can define computational modelling as the simulation of a computational theory or part of that theory. This activity goes beyond appealing to some kind of computational metaphor as part of a psychological theory and *implements* at least a fragment of a theory as a *simulation* of an aspect of intelligent behaviour.

Computational modelling has a number of uses within theory development in cognitive psychology and cognitive neuropsychology. First, the activity can help make some rather vague ideas clearer. Having to implement a model as a computer simulation forces the modeller to be explicit, both in how information is represented and in the way it is processed. Theoretical claims have to become concrete enough to be expressed as parts of a computer program. Additionally, implementing a model is a good way of checking that its claims are internally consistent. If they are not then the model won't work or will operate in unexpected ways.

Modelling allows the exploration of complex ideas and parameters. It is not always easy to grasp how complex models will operate without expressing them as a simulation. McClelland (1988) gives an example of this advantage of modelling in his discussion of the work that was stimulated by the McClelland and Rumelhart (1981) model of visual word perception.

When simulating semantic processing, the modeller is forced to think hard about the representational assumptions that are being used. As we shall see at the end of the chapter, once a neural network has learned about several objects encoded as feature-based semantic representations, it can display category specificity even though the items stored have not been labelled by category. Computational modelling has become particularly important in cognitive neuropsychology since when a concrete implementation of a cognitive system is damaged it is possible to explore whether the damaged system performs like a person with brain damage.

Finally, computational modelling often allows us to make novel predictions. One of the properties of a good theory is that it makes novel, testable predictions. Computational models allow parameters to be manipulated to give explicit, often quantitative predictions.

Computational modelling also has certain disadvantages and dangers. There can be a difficulty in ensuring that a model transparently implements aspects of a theory. There is always a degree of abstraction and compromise when theories are implemented as models. A model exists within a particular system defined by a particular simulation program or programming language. The need to use explicit representations may mean that some aspects of the original theory have to be simplified, e.g. what constitutes a realistic semantic representation. Some of these problems might be mitigated as computational principles become more and more integrated within mainstream cognitive theory. If theories are stated in terms that more closely correspond to concrete computation then their implementation is bound to be more transparent, though there is perhaps a danger of circularity here.

One of the compromises often made in modelling a cognitive phenomenon is to simplify the scale of the problem: e.g. by limiting the size of a memory or the number of phonemes used in an input representation of the sound of a word. The modeller must be able to claim that their simulation is capable in principle of being extended to a realistic size.

Certain models and frameworks are so expressive or computationally powerful that they can be made to mimic virtually any result. Their operation must take place within psychologically relevant constraints if any advance in explanation is to be made.

Finally, there is little to be gained by merely simulating a phenomenon if it is unclear how the simulation works or the simulation merely restates a clearly formulated theory and does nothing to extend it or produce novel hypotheses.

A good computational model gives a clear account of some data or a particular theoretical idea. It should have advantages compared to a linguistic or static mathematical exposition of a theory. It should produce novel predictions and constrained behaviour. Ideally, a model should be capable of simulating a task at full scale. Models should stimulate theoretical debate and development even if they are shown to be wrong.

The attractions of connectionism

Connectionism is the usual term for a particular biologically inspired form of computational modelling which has special attractions for cognitive modelling. In outlining the main characteristics of connectionist networks and how they operate, the chapter will use the terms connectionist network, neural network and parallel distributed processing (PDP) network interchangeably.

Neural networks are made up from simple units connected by weighted connections. In sharp comparison to the powerful, all-purpose processors used in symbolic systems, the units in neural networks are very simple devices. Their behaviour depends on the excitation or inhibition they receive either directly or via connections from other units. An item such as a word or concept is often represented as a pattern of active units that can cause another pattern to occur when activation spreads. The way the activation spreads depends on the balance of weights between the units.

The systems can learn by changing the weights to appropriate values. Regularities can be learned automatically and do not have to be specified beforehand by the modeller. Neural networks have many psychologically interesting basic properties like the ability to learn rules and exceptions, content addressability, noise resistance, graceful degradation and the ability to map one level of representation to another. These properties are explained below. They can display complex dynamics in the way that activation flows through them. Many of the interesting computational properties of neural nets depend on the way that the patterns of activation change across time. The systems can be damaged and used as models of cognitive neuropsychology. This trades on the supposed 'brain style' computation of neural nets as well as some of their natural properties such as distribution, graceful degradation and noise tolerance.

General attractions for cognitive modelling

What computational properties make connectionist networks so attractive for cognitive modelling? This chapter will now briefly describe some of these abilities before going on to outline how these properties arise from the details of neural network functioning. Their processing of information can be said to occur *in parallel*. Whole patterns of activation can be dealt with at one time because many units can be active at the same time.

Some of the most striking properties of neural networks include content addressability and pattern completion. These phenomena occur when the input of part of a pattern leads to retrieval of the rest. This natural property of networks that have *point attractors* in their dynamics is compellingly similar to some of the properties of human memory. There is no external process searching through the memory but instead active memory patterns that can settle into a state that represents stored knowledge when constrained with a partial cue. Noise resistance and graceful degradation are related properties. A certain amount of input noise or structural damage can be tolerated. This is partly due to distributed representations and connections that may contain a degree of redundancy and partly a by-product of the same processes that underlie content addressability. The best solution to multiple constraints is reached and this can still be a fairly good solution if some constraints are faulty or missing.

It is not hard to see how a neural network can map between one class of representations and another. This is a natural consequence of the way that units can be arranged in layers and the weights between them set so that a class of patterns on one layer tends to cause the activation of a second class of patterns on another layer.

There are several ways that allow the networks to learn patterns or classes of patterns. These learning algorithms are methods of specifying the appropriate combination of weights between the units in the network to cause the correct pattern of activation to flow through the network. Under certain circumstances this allows these systems to build their own internal representations that mediate the mapping between one level of structure and another.

Neural networks confound process and representation. The processing and representation within the network are both entirely controlled by the weights. The representations can be seen as active and weights can be construed as constraints on the way that activation spreads. Sub-symbolic or distributed information is represented as diffuse patterns of activation rather than discrete symbols.

As mentioned above, there has been a great deal of recent research on the use of connectionism to model cognitive neuropsychological phenomena. It is easy to damage a connectionist network to explore the predictions of a cognitive neuropsychological theory. There are several different ways of 'lesioning' a network, e.g. units or weights can be removed or noise added to the unit activations. Damage can be gradual and graded. There is a natural way to model a lack of general cognitive resources. This can be achieved by reducing the number of hidden units available during learning. It is possible to model different strategies for the rehabilitation of people with neuropsychological deficits by damaging a network and looking at different schemes for retraining it (see Plaut, 1992; 1996).

How do neural networks work?

The basic properties of connectionist computation are as follows. A neural network is made up of simple units each connected to many others. Each connection carries a weight and the effect of one unit on another is determined by the strength of the weight: the effects can be excitatory if positive or inhibitory if negative, and of differing strengths. When information is fed into a connectionist system, a pattern of activation spreads through the network. Activation can spread in one direction only or the system can have complex dynamics with feedback. Several patterns can be stored, superimposed in the same weights. Certain architectures can give rise to stable states or patterns. This is the property that leads to content address-ability, noise resistance, etc. In a layered network, the input layer can represent one level of representation and the output layer a second level. The network can then be seen to function as a method of mapping between the two levels. Learning algorithms are methods of adjusting the weights so that the network stores the right patterns or performs the right mapping. The weights can be seen as constraints and the learning process as a way of finding the right balance of constraints.

There are occasions where information in a neural network is repre-sented in a local fashion, i.e. individual units stand for particular items. However, many of the attractive qualities of connectionism arise from distributed representation where each item, idea, concept or whatever is represented by a distributed pattern of representation across a number of different units. Different items are represented by different patterns across the same units. The individual unit activations may not have a semantic interpretation or they may correspond to the presence or absence of a 'microfeature'. The similarity between two items is repre-sented by the similarity in the patterns of activation that represent them. In the appropriate system, this allows the network to come up with novel outputs based on *generalizations* from the inputs it has been trained on. Distributed representations tend to be robust or noise resistant. Sometimes it is convenient for a particular model to use a relatively localist representation. For example, the lexical entry for a word is often represented as a single labelled unit (McClelland and Elman, 1986). The advantages of distributed representation are being traded for conve-nience and the fact that we are largely ignorant of how to represent much of the information that would go into making a distributed lexical repre-sentation.

Information is fed into a network using input units and read off from output units. Minsky and Papert (1969) showed that simple two-layered networks were incapable of performing some quite basic computations. One example of such a computation is the XOR or parity function. It is impossible to set the weights for a 2 input unit and one output unit network in such a way that the output is 1 if either input unit is 1 but the output is 0 if both inputs are 0 or both units are 1. This kind of function requires an extra unit or in the general case a layer of extra units. The extra units are not input or output units and are thus called hidden units. Hidden units act as ways of separating out similar input patterns. They can be seen as internal representations within the network.

Most people would agree that one of the advantages of connectionism is that it supports 'brain-style' computation. The degree of biological realism that is thought to be important varies widely: from a level where neurophysiology and psychology merge, to one where units and connections are mere metaphors. It is certainly the case that most connectionist cognitive models contain some aspects that are biologically implausible. One example is that synapses are either excitatory or inhibitory and yet learning algorithms often allow weights to change from positive to negative or vice versa.

Semantic representations in connectionist models

There are various ways in which semantic information can be represented in connectionist models.

Some research has taken advantage of explicit human judgements. For example, participants can be asked to generate a set of properties for a group of words (McRae, deSa, and Seidenberg 1993; 1997). Each consistently used property can then be used as a dimension in the vector space expressed as the activation of a particular unit in a connectionist network. The advantage of this approach is that the data are generated from genuine human judgements and hence have some kind of psychological validity. One disadvantage is that participants probably employ particular strategies when asked to generate such information. They are likely to volunteer more specific distinguishing features than information that is shared within a group and so not distinguishing. Thus the properties generated may reflect what is thought to be informative rather than what truly underlies semantic knowledge. Another more practical disadvantage is that the technique is laborious and small scale, requiring a large number of participants to generate vectors for a relatively small number of target words.

Another approach is for the experimenters or modellers to generate the semantic vector space themselves using their personal intuition

(Hinton and Shallice, 1991; Plaut and Shallice, 1993). The advantage of this approach is that the proposed representational structures can be specified simply and directly. For example, Plaut and Shallice chose an intuitively plausible micro-feature representation in which concrete entities were specified by more micro-features than abstract entities. A concrete word like *lass* would have 20 micro-features including 'main-shape-3D', 'soft', 'human' and 'female'. An abstract word like *loss* would have only four: 'negative', 'involves-change', 'future-potential' and 'relates-money'. The disadvantage here is the lack of external validation. When Plaut and Shallice make claims about the differences between concrete and abstract words they are open to the attack that they themselves have built the differences into their semantic feature representations.

A third method has been to use randomly generated vectors. Some modellers argue that for purposes of simulating the essentially arbitrary mapping between mono-morphemic phonology/orthography and semantics, a random semantic vector space is sufficient to capture the essential effects (Bullinaria, 1995; Plaut, 1995). Others have used a random semantic space as a placeholder with a semantic lexicon to reflect the fact that, say, phonology and semantics occur at the same level but have not yet reached a point where their modelling needs the details of the semantics to be specified (Gaskell and Marslen-Wilson, 1997). This approach has the advantage of simplicity and external validity as long as the details of the semantic structure do not play a role in the processes being modelled. The disadvantage is that there is no way of modelling how semantic structure might have a role.

A fourth method that has recently been used is to use WordNet (Fellbaum, 1998), a lexicographical database, to specify a word's semantic features (Patel, 1996; Harm, 1998). The approach has external validation from the intuition of the linguists who constructed the database. However, WordNet is not adequate for all word types (Harm, 1998) and linguists' intuitions do not necessarily reflect underlying mental representations.

Recent work in computational and cognitive psychology (Landauer and Dumais, 1997; Levy, Bullinaria and Patel, 1998) has shown that some interesting aspects of the properties of a word can be captured by simple statistical counts of which other words tend to occur close to the target word.

An example might be to take a large text corpus and for each word (target) in it count the number of times each other word type occurs within a window of, say, 10 words. After the counting exercise, each word is represented as a vector consisting of the cumulative frequencies of occurrence of each word type within the window. For a particular word, its resulting vector represents the kind of verbal environment it tends to occur in. If the technique works, words with similar meanings will tend to occur in similar contexts and hence have vectors that largely overlap or are close in vector space. This kind of pattern of usage may prove to be a useful representation of lexical semantics for cognitive modelling. It has the advantages of using real language use as its raw material and being able to generate a representation of any word of reasonably high frequency. It has the disadvantages of being purely verbal and instantiating only a shallow reflection of word meaning as pattern of use.

Connectionist models of semantic category-specific deficits

A number of recent connectionist models explore different claims about the nature of category-specific deficits (see Chapter 4). Such models test representational assumptions by explicitly formulating patterns for living things and man-made artefacts that accord with the assumptions, and by examining how behaviour breaks down following damage to networks trained on the patterns. They claim that category-specific deficits need not arise from localization of category information. Farah and McClelland (1991) suggest that the deficits are due to differences in the functional and perceptual information balance between categories and specific damage to functional or perceptual information (see Chapter 1). Other models make claims about details of the internal structure of the semantic representation that do not rely on localized damage.

Warrington and colleagues (Warrington and McCarthy, 1983; Warrington and Shallice, 1984) suggested that semantic category deficits are due to differential damage to perceptual and functional information. (We shall see that future workers in this field have sought to explore what exactly is meant by 'functional' information). They claimed that living things are predominantly distinguished by their sensory properties and man-made things by their function or what they are used for. Thus if perceptual information is degraded or lost then there will be a differential loss of knowledge about living things, with the reverse dissociation occurring for loss of functional attributes.

This 'perceptual-functional' argument can also explain observations where dissociations don't neatly fall across the living/non-living distinction. Warrington and Shallice's (1984) observation of a living thing's deficit accompanied by impaired knowledge of fabrics and gemstones can be explained by these categories having primarily perceptual properties unlike most man-made artefacts. Similarly, the behaviour of the person observed by Warrington and McCarthy (1987), who had a general artefact deficit but with spared knowledge of large outdoor objects like bridges and windmills, can be explained if these objects have a predominantly visual representation.

Farah and McClelland (1991)

Farah and McClelland report an important model that tested these ideas and demonstrated that implementing them extended the explanation beyond what could have been expected from the simple verbal description of the perceptual-functional distinction. It illustrates how the activity of modelling a theoretical viewpoint can yield benefits beyond a simple confirmation of the original ideas. Since their model paved the way for subsequent work it is examined in some detail here.

Farah and McClelland began by testing the perceptual–functional distinction. They asked normal participants to underline visual and functional descriptors in dictionary definitions of living and non-living things. Separate groups of participants checked for perceptual (visual) and functional descriptors. The participants reading for perceptual descriptors underlined an average of 2.68 for living things and 1.57 for non-living things. The other group of participants underlined an average of 0.35 functional features for living things and 1.11 for non-living things. The experiment thus confirmed the hypothesis that visual descriptors are particularly important for living things: there was an average ratio of 7.7:1 of visual features to functional features for living things and 1.4:1 for non-living things. Functional features are less important for living things than they are for non-living things (at least in relation to their number) but the experiment found that there were still 40% more visual features than functional features for non-living things. So, although functional features are relatively more important for non-living things than they are for living things, Farah and McClelland based their model on their observation that perceptual features outnumbered functional features for both living and non-living domains with only the degree of the ratio differentiating them. The average ratio of perceptual to functional descriptors across both living and non-living things was 2.9:1.

Farah and McClelland wanted to model data from people with brain damage who had been tested on picture-naming and matching-to-sample tasks. They structured their model with this purpose in mind. The network contained three pools of units: verbal input/output units, visual input/output units and, connected in between the two pools of input/output units, 80 semantic memory units. The semantic memory units were made up from 60 visual units and 20 functional units. This 3:1 ratio of visual to functional units corresponded to the average proportion observed in the dictionary entry rating exercise. The random activations of the verbal units stood for the name of a particular item. The activations of the visual input/output units stood for attributes of pictures of the items. The memory units represented the pattern of perceptual and functional information that forms the basis for the long-term knowledge about each living and non-living item.

The units were allowed to take on activation values of between –1 and +1. Both the name and the picture unit pool were bi-directionally connected to all the semantic units. All the units within each pool were bi-directionally connected to each other. This allows the network to have dynamic behaviour whereby it can gradually 'settle' into a stable state after the weights have been set appropriately by a learning algorithm.

Representations of 10 living and 10 non-living things were generated randomly except for a number of constraints to reflect the aspects of semantic structure that were being modelled. All units in the three pools were set to either +1 or –1 except some of the semantic units that were unused and so set to zero. For each item, all the name and picture units were used but only a subset of the semantic units were set to +1 or –1 to reflect the differential importance of perceptual and semantic information for the living and non-living domains. For living things an average 16.1 visual units and 2.1 functional units were used (a ratio of 7.7:1). For non-living things an average of 9.4 visual and 6.7 functional units were used (a ratio of 1.4:1).

The purpose of the model was to simulate how picture naming and matching-to-sample break down when the trained network is damaged. The network was trained with these aims in mind. The weights between the units were set so that each of the 20 items was a stable state in the dynamics of the network. This was achieved by using a simple delta learning rule. Back propagation was not required since there were no hidden units.

There were two configurations of training that reflected the two activities that the network was to carry out. To ensure that the network could simulate picture naming, the picture pattern for an item was presented to the visual units and the network allowed to settle for 10 cycles. The delta rule was then used to adjust all the weights so that the error between the target values and the actual values was reduced for the semantic memory units and the name units for the item being trained. This operation was done in reverse to train the network for matching a picture to a name by presenting a pattern on the name units and adjusting the weights so that the semantic memory units and picture units became closer to their targets. Both operations were repeated for each of the 20 items for 100 training epochs. Farah and McClelland used a trick of the modelling trade to make the network more resistant to damage. They employed a technique called *weight decay* where each weight is reduced slightly at the end of each training epoch.

At the end of training the network was able to simulate both naming and matching-to-sample tasks. The model could be used to associate the name and picture units via the semantic units. Picture naming was simulated by imposing a pattern on the picture units and then seeing what pattern appeared on the name units after settling, and picture selection was simulated by imposing a pattern on the name units and watching the picture units settle. The network was capable of this because all the weights were set appropriately so that interaction between units within each pool and between the pools contributed to each response. It is this distribution of activity as well as the distributed patterns of representation that were used to explain the patterns of behaviour after the network was lesioned.

Farah and McClelland used four different versions of their model but since most of their results applied to all the versions we shall examine the basic model only. The model simulates category-specific deficits by damaging either the functional or visual aspects of semantic memory. There are several different ways in which this kind of damage could have been inflicted on the network, including adding noise to the network or damaging network connections. Farah and McClelland chose to set a probability with which a particular visual or functional unit would be destroyed.

The network was 'lesioned' by uniformly damaging either the visual or the functional semantic memory units with a given probability (0%, 20%, 40%, 60%, 80% or 99%). At each separate level of damage all 20 items were tested in a simulation of a picture-naming task and a simulation of a matching-to-sample task. Each of the 40 trials was scored correct if the output pattern was closer to the target activation than any of the other 19 other outputs.

The results displayed a clear category-specific effect. When the visual semantic memory units were damaged performance on non-living items declined slowly to a level of around 70% correct when all the visual semantic units had been destroyed. Performance on living things declined much more quickly showing a greater deficit than for non-living things at 40% damage and declining to almost zero when all the visual semantic units had been lesioned.

When the functional semantic memory units were damaged the reverse dissociation occurred but was less extreme. Performance on living things was perfect even when all the functional semantic units were destroyed. After 20% of these units had been destroyed, performance on non-living things dropped slowly to a level of around 70% when all the functional units had been lesioned.

The observed dissociations confirm the theoretical principles that were used to build the network model. Damaging the visual semantic features affects the living things items more than the non-living items because the semantic representation of living things is predominantly made up of visual features. However, the non-living items still suffer a deficit in performance because they do contain a few visual features. Damaging the functional semantic features doesn't affect the living things items at all since their semantic representation depends overwhelmingly on perceptual features. Damaged functional units had a marked but not catastrophic effect on non-living things, reflecting the fact that functional information was important in their representation but perceptual information still made up more than half the number of specified features in each non-living item semantic memory pattern.

Farah and McClelland then went on to demonstrate that their model could account for data from early studies of category-specific deficits (Silveri and Gainotti, 1988; Basso, Capitani, and Laiacona, 1988) that showed a living things deficit accompanied by both loss of perceptual knowledge of living things and loss of functional knowledge. This appears to be problematic for the perceptual-functional hypothesis since it implies that specific perceptual and functional damage is required to account for a living things deficit.

Farah and McClelland demonstrated this effect by training and lesioning the network as before but measuring an average error across the functional or perceptual units. They used a method of getting an error measure that compares the whole pattern of unit activations with the appropriate target pattern. This was achieved by calculating the average dot products between the actual functional or perceptual unit patterns and their respective targets, normalized to 1 for the undamaged network. The data demonstrated that when visual semantic units were damaged living things lost both this perceptual knowledge and, to a marked extent, lost functional information as well. Functional semantic memory for non-living things was less strongly affected by damaging the visual semantic units.

The loss of both perceptual and functional semantic knowledge for living things when only perceptual units were directly damaged may be explained by reference to the properties of distributed representations in neural networks. The activation of each unit is supported by connections from the other units participating in a pattern. There may be a kind of 'critical mass' effect whereby if enough of the other units in a pattern are damaged then an undamaged unit may perhaps not receive the correct support and so will have an incorrect activation value. This may happen for the functional units for living things when several perceptual units are damaged. The effect doesn't occur for non-living things because their representations are more predominantly functional and so functional units can provide mutual support when perceptual units are damaged.

Finally, Farah and McClelland used their network to model the person described by McCarthy and Warrington (1988) who displayed a living things deficit only when tested verbally. He was impaired at defining living things when they were named aloud. This pattern of behaviour appears to suggest that semantic knowledge is duplicated depending on whether it is to be accessed by visual or verbal means. In fact, this data could be simulated without the use of different stores by damaging the connections between the name units and the visual semantics units. When these connections were damaged at increasing levels there was no deficit in producing a name pattern in response to a picture pattern. There was some impairment in producing a picture pattern of a non-living thing in response to a name pattern but there was sharply decreasing performance when the task of the network was to produce a picture pattern for a living thing in response to a name. Thus, the network produced a category- and modality-specific deficit by damaging the route from names to semantic memory in a system with a unitary semantic store.

Farah and McClelland's model successfully demonstrated the internal consistency of the perceptual-functional hypothesis by implementing a system that, when damaged in a modality-specific manner, displayed both major kinds of category-specific deficit. Furthermore, because the network acted as a distributed memory system, it showed why damaging perceptual semantic memory units caused functional knowledge deficits in living things by disrupting the usual support that perceptual units gave to functional units. Finally, they showed that their system could simulate a modality- and category-specific effect when one particular route into semantic memory was damaged. As a result the way was paved for subsequent work that explored further assumptions about how different representational schemes might give rise to category-specific deficits.

Small, Hart, Nguyen and Gordon (1995)

Small et al. (1995) presented computational simulations and mathematical analyses that demonstrated how category specificity could emerge from the nature of semantic features rather than any internal categorical organization.

Using two different kinds of representation, Small et al. constructed two different kinds of network in order to analyse how categories might emerge from the interaction of semantic features in a connectionist network. The first kind of representation was a simple one-unit-per-item object representation where an item was identified by which output unit (out of 57) was most active. The second kind of representation was an array of 77 semantic features that were either true or false of an object. The features described aspects of the physical appearance of an object (e.g. how many legs, which colour), other perceptual attributes such as the noise the object makes, motor associations (e.g. whether self-moving) and functional information (e.g. purpose of a tool, biological activities such as reproduction or producing waste).

The first network architecture was a simple two-layer associator network where the semantic feature values on the input layer were mapped on to 57 object identification units using a delta learning rule. The second network was an 'autoassociator' where the 77 semantic feature values were used as input and activation flowed through two hidden layers to recreate the semantic feature unit activations on the output layer. This network was trained using back propagation.

Small et al. used five different techniques to analyse the representations used by the networks including the hidden unit activations that the network developed during learning as well as the pre-coded ones imposed on the input and output layers. Using methods such as cluster analysis, competitive learning and principal components analysis they showed how their feature-based descriptions of objects implicitly embodied category information. The categories found by these methods were not perfect or clear-cut but rather reflected the imprecise nature of real-life category boundaries. Importantly, the category structure emerged from the similarities between the different feature patterns since there was no explicit information about category in the feature representations.

An example of the analytic techniques used by Small et al. was their use of principal components analysis on the patterns of activation on the second hidden layer of the autoassociator network. Principal components analysis summarizes the most important dimensions of variation in a set of patterns. They found principal components that appeared to code for animals and hand tools as well as one that effectively distinguished living from non-living things. They thus demonstrated that a set of features that had been chosen to effectively describe a set of 57 objects could yield several kinds of categorical information when learned by a neural network.

In their discussion of category-specific deficits, Small et al. point out that if semantic information is represented in the brain in a manner similar to their feature-based networks then the distributedness of the information leads to robustness and non-localization of categorization ability. This accounts for the rarity of category-specific deficits and the difficulty (or impossibility) of discovering the neurological localization of categories. However, the authors do not attempt to give an explanation of specific dissociations or double dissociations of different categories. Subsequent modelling by other workers has explored some of the consequences of more specific assumptions in feature structure.

Devlin, Gonnerman, Andersen, and Seidenberg (1998)

Devlin et al. (1998) describe a model of the category-specific deficits observed in people with Alzheimer's disease (AD; see also Chapter 7). This condition is progressive and the cortical damage is rather diffuse in contrast to the acute and rather focal damage caused by herpes simplex encephalitis (HSE) which is the condition associated with many category-specific deficits. Devlin et al. describe a model that extends the work of Gonnerman, Andersen, Devlin et al. (1997) who explained the category-specific deficits that they observed in people with AD in terms of progressive damage to a unitary semantic system where living things were more intercorrelated and had less distinctive features than was the case for artefacts.

Devlin et al. aimed to model the AD data as random damage to a single semantic system as well as replicating the results of Farah and McClelland (1991) who showed how focal damage to functional or perceptual information could cause the kind of category-specific deficit found in HSE. Their model of the AD data doesn't depend on the proportion of functional or perceptual information associated with different kinds of category as was the case in Farah and McClelland (1991). They claim on the basis of empirical data that living things and artefacts differ in the internal organization of semantic features. They simulate the consequences of random progressive damage on such representations.

Following McRae, deSa, and Seidenberg (1993 – see also McRae et al., 1997), Devlin et al. use property norms as the source of the semantic features in their network model. McRae et al. demonstrated the importance of intercorrelations between properties in accounting for semantic priming data. Devlin et al. also stress the varying importance or distinctiveness of different properties. The more distinctive a property or feature is the more it distinguishes one individual item from another within a category.

The model is based on property norms collected from 30 undergraduate participants. They were asked to list the perceptual and functional properties of 60 items, 30 living things and 30 artefacts. The living things were made up from 15 fruits and vegetables and 15 animals. The artefacts were made up from 10 vehicles, 10 items of clothing and 10 tools. The most popular 145 properties were used as binary features in the semantic representations of the network model. Of these features, 88 were perceptual and 57 were functional.

Like Farah and McClelland (1991), they found that, on average, all items had more perceptual properties than functional properties but that this ratio was higher for living things. Following McRae et al. (1993), they calculated the correlation coefficients for all the combinations of feature pairs. Of these statistics 416 were significant. Living things had a mean of 18.3 significant correlations while artefacts had a mean of 13.8. The natural consequence of this is that living things share more properties within a category than do artefacts. This means that, on average, a particular feature in the representation of a living thing is less distinctive and so less informative in identifying an item than is the case of a property of an artefact. From this it follows that random damage is more likely to cause confusion in identifying individual artefact items while the representations of living things will be more robust in this respect.

Gonnerman et al. (1997) claimed that this tendency to fragility in artefact representations would cause an artefact deficit with moderate diffuse damage to the representations. Later in the course of a progressive but patchy condition like AD, so many properties would be lost that the intercorrelations that support the shared properties of living things would be lost and this would cause a catastrophic living things deficit. Without as much dependence on intercorrelative category structure, artefacts would suffer a more gradual decrease in performance as individual properties were lost.

The model of Devlin et al. was constructed in order to model the mapping between a semantic level of representation and a phonological level. The phonological patterns for each of the 60 words were random patterns of 40 features with a mean of 12.9 active features. The representations were random because the modellers wanted the mapping between semantics and phonology to be a completely arbitrary one (although this would still have been the case if the phonology alone had been structured).

The network model consisted of the pool of semantic units bi-directionally connected to the pool of phonology units. The semantic units were also bi-directionally connected to 20 clean-up units and the phonology pool had 8 clean-up units. The clean-up units helped support the memory of each of the 60 items as a stable state or attractor in the dynamics of the semantic and phonological representations after training.

Presenting a semantic pattern and allowing the network to settle to produce a phonological output simulated the production of a word. The reverse process where a phonological pattern was used as input and a semantic pattern produced as output simulated language comprehension.

The network was trained using a version of the back propagation learning algorithm that was capable of taking the feedback or recurrence of the network into account. Each of the 60 items was presented as a semantic pattern and the weights changed so that when the network settled the appropriate pattern was instantiated on the phonological units. This was also performed in reverse so that each of the 60 phonological patterns produced the correct pattern of semantic features. The end result was that the joint phonological-semantic pattern for each item was a stable state or point attractor in the dynamics of the network and so presenting one part of the pattern caused the other part to become activated.

After the network was successfully trained, Devlin et al. damaged it to simulate the effect of Alzheimer's disease on the semantic representations. They chose to mimic the kind of damage inflicted by AD by randomly removing connections within the semantic system of the network. The progressive nature of AD damage was simulated by progressively lesioning the network connections. First, 1% of the connections were removed at a time and then after 20% had been removed, 5% were removed at a time and then 10% lesions were made after 50% of the connections had been removed. The process was repeated on 50 networks to simulate 50 different network 'participants'.

The different networks showed a variety of interesting patterns of deficit. The average results showed a living things deficit that worsened as damage accumulated to the networks. However, this pattern was in fact made up of two major sub-patterns. The most frequent pattern occurred with 38 of the 50 simulations. Here, there was an initial mild artefact deficit that became an increasingly severe living things deficit after about 20% damage. In a further 11 of the simulations there was a living things deficit that progressively worsened right from the start. Within these sub-patterns there was a large degree of variation in the behaviour of individual simulations. There was a remaining individual simulation where an initial living things deficit became an artefacts deficit and then a severe global deficit.

So, in over three-quarters of the individual simulations, Devlin et al.'s predicted behaviour was borne out. There was an initial artefact deficit caused by sporadic loss of vital distinctive semantic features followed by a living things deficit caused by increasingly severe collapse of the shared features that underpin living things categories. However, this was not the case for all of the damaged networks.

Devlin et al. also replicated the basic result of Farah and McClelland (1991) by focally lesioning either the perceptual or functional features within the semantic pool of units and obtaining a living things deficit and an artefact deficit respectively.

The Devlin et al. model extends previous work to show that, as well as a double dissociation between living and non-living things caused by differential damage to perceptual and functional features, progressive diffuse damage can also produce category-specific deficits. Using damage designed to mimic the characteristics of AD they showed that a kind of chronological double dissociation occurs in most of their simulations. An initially mild artefacts deficit 'crosses over' into a progressively worsening living things deficit. These dissociations don't reflect any modularity within the semantic system but rather a difference in the pattern of property distinctiveness and co-occurrences between different semantic categories. It would have been very difficult to demonstrate the consequences of such semantic structure without modelling it in different connectionist networks.

Durrant-Peatfield, Tyler, Moss and Levy (1997)

Durrant-Peatfield et al. (1997) describe another representational scheme that produces category-specific deficits when damaged randomly and diffusely. They emphasize the importance of functional information in semantic representation and make claims about how living things and artefacts differ in the way they make use of functional information and the way it is correlated with perceptual information. They point to evidence for the salience and robustness of functional information (Moss, Tyler, Hodges et al., 1995; Moss, Tyler, Durrant-Peatfield et al., 1996; Tyler and Moss, 1997).

Durrant-Peatfield et al. claim that for most artefacts functional information is distinctive and is strongly correlated with the perceptual information that describes that part of the artefact that performs its designed function, e.g. a knife's function of cutting is correlated with the visual attributes of a blade. Usually, what distinguishes living things from each other is perceptual information and this is not correlated with any functional information, e.g. the stripes of a zebra. The representation of a living thing does contain functional information in the form of biological function, the function of the different mechanisms that allow a living thing to operate, such as eyes for vision and lungs for breathing. Biological functional information is highly correlated with perceptual information but is not distinctive. It makes up part of the densely intercorrelated category information described by Devlin et al.

Durrant-Peatfield at al. constructed some feature patterns to test these ideas. Living things are distinguished by uncorrelated perceptual features and have dense intercorrelated biological function and non-distinctive perceptual information. Artefacts are distinguished by strongly correlated perceptual-functional feature pairs but do not have as well supported shared category structure. Sixteen patterns of 24 features represented two groups of four living things and two groups of four artefacts.

The patterns were used to construct a three-layer connectionist network where the 24 feature values on an input layer were reconstructed on an identical output layer via a hidden layer. The weights were trained using the back propagation learning algorithm.

After the network had been trained it was lesioned by removing different proportions of the weights between 10% and 80% in 10% increments. The process was repeated for 300 different networks. They found that the distinctive features for living things were more prone to damage than the strongly correlated distinctive features for artefacts. This artefact advantage tended to be reversed after about 60% of the weights had been lesioned. Shared information was uniformly more robust for living things than for artefacts.

After lesioning, each pattern was compared to all 24 of the original patterns and matched to the closest corresponding pattern. The errors observed for the individual kinds of features were reflected in the overall classification performance and the between- and within-category errors observed at the level of whole patterns. There was an overall living things deficit until around 60% of the weights had been removed where there was a cross-over to an artefacts deficit. Performance on living things was particularly characterized by a large proportion of within-category errors where a pattern was confused for another within the correct category. This is what would be expected from a loss of distinctive features with spared shared category structure. Artefacts were more prone to between-category errors than was the case for living things. This reflects the relatively unsupported shared information within the artefact categories.

The model of Durrant-Peatfield et al. predicts that diffuse damage to the kind of representation that they build into their model will produce a deficit where living things are confused between each other but where both artefact functional and biological functional information is relatively spared. They claim that this is indeed what is found in people, citing RC (Moss et al., 1996) who suffered a living things deficit after HSE. The network model also predicts that the relatively rare artefact deficit may occur after very severe damage to such a system.

Recent models

French and Mareschal (1998) suggest another way in which differences in the underlying representations of living things and artefacts may cause category-specific deficits when a unitary semantic store is damaged. They claim that categories differ in their variability and that this makes them differ in their vulnerability to damage.

They simulated an autoassociator network that learned 20 patterns that represented the physical attributes of chairs and 20 that represented different butterflies. They observed that the representations of chairs were more variable than those of butterflies. This makes the hidden unit representations of butterflies more compact and hence more prone to disruption by random damage to the network. This is indeed what they found. In most of the simulations there was a living things deficit. However, in about 10% of cases the reverse dissociation was found.

French and Mareschal's model illustrates another way to describe how category structure can vary and hence display a disparity after damage.

Zorzi, Perry, Ziegler et al. (1999) claim that the basis of semantic category organization in the brain lies at an abstract 'lemma' level. This is then mapped on to other levels of knowledge such as visual features or phonology. They model the lemma level as a topographically organized 'self-organized' map. This is a kind of neural network that can spontaneously group similar objects together without any kind of external supervision. If objects are described as either possessing or not possessing a variety of features, then a self-organizing map can be visualized as a collapsed two-dimensional space that preserves the important categorical organization of the objects. Similar objects cluster together into groups that correspond to categories.

Zorzi et al. model category-specific deficits by damaging some of the nodes in the map. This produced dramatic category-specific deficits of different kinds depending on which nodes were damaged. Their results are preliminary and they have yet to give a detailed description of their simulations. Their model shows how focal lesions may cause category-specific deficits by removing important information about a category that has become locally represented in a semantic map.

Conclusion

The idea that category specificity need not imply localization of category information is one where connectionist modelling has proved its worth. The models described here make different claims about how different kinds of information or different characteristics of how information is internally related can account for category specificity. We can confirm the basic coherence of these ideas by implementing them as neural networks and then damaging them. This allows us to explore the various claims in ways that would be impossible without some kind of simulation.

Most neural network models aren't completely biologically realistic but they do embody enough of what we know about 'brain style computation' to add explanatory weight to simulations of theoretical ideas.

The simulations described here all display category-specific deficits of various different kinds. Their claims are not necessarily mutually exclusive. However, future progress with this kind of modelling must surely lie with closer attention to specific clinical data and the gaining of a more secure foundation for the origin of semantic representations. For example, we need to know more securely the conditions under which artefact deficits are found. Devlin at al. and Durrant-Peatfield et al. make different predictions about how much damage needs to be done to the semantic representation for an artefact deficit to occur. Whether these are contradictory depends on whether artefact deficits can arise from different kinds of brain damage.

More clinical data and modern techniques such as functional imaging will allow the models discussed here to be tested by giving further insight into the following questions, among others:

- Are category-specific deficits due to damage to modality-specific brain systems or unitary semantic systems or both?
- How exactly do damage from HSE and damage from AD differ and how is this manifested in semantic deficits?
- What is the range of individual differences in response to different categories of damage?
- Under what conditions are artefact deficits found?

Connectionist models are not a panacea for theories about the cognitive neuropsychology of semantics. However, they do offer a framework for understanding how theoretical claims about the organization of knowledge stand up to an explicit computational test.

References

Basso A, Capitani E, Laiacona M (1988) Progressive language impairment without dementia: a case with isolated category-specific semantic deficit. Journal of Neurology, Neurosurgery and Psychiatry 51: 1201–07.

Bullinaria JA (1995) Modelling lexical decision: Who needs a lexicon? In Keating JG, (Ed) Neural computing research and applications III. Maynooth, Ireland: St Patrick's College. pp 62–69.

Devlin JT, Gonnerman L, Andersen E, Seidenberg M (1998) Category specific deficits in focal and widespread damage: a computational account. Journal of Cognitive Neuroscience 10(1): 77–94.

Durrant-Peatfield M, Tyler LK, Moss H, Levy JP (1997) The distinctiveness of form and function in category structure: a connectionist model. In Shafto MG, Langley P, (Eds) Proceedings of the 19th Annual Conference of the Cognitive Science Society. Mahwah, NJ: LEA. pp 193–98.

Farah MJ, McClelland JL (1991) A computational model of semantic impairment: modality specificity and emergent category specificity. Journal of Experimental Psychology: General 120(4): 339–57.

Fellbaum C, (Ed) (1998) WordNet: An electronic lexical database. Cambridge, MA: MIT Press.

French RM, Mareschal D (1988) Could category-specific semantic deficits reflect differences in the distributions of features within a unified semantic memory? In

Proceedings of the 20th Annual Conference of the Cognitive Science Society. NJ: LEA. pp 374–79.

Gaskell G, Marslen-Wilson W (1997) Discriminating local and distributed models of competition in spoken word recognition. In Shafto MG, Langley P, (Eds) Proceedings of the 19th Annual Conference of the Cognitive Science Society. Mahwah, NJ: LEA. pp 247–52.

Gonnerman LM, Andersen ES, Devlin JT, Kempler D, Seidenberg M (1997) Double dissociation of semantic categories in Alzheimer's disease. Brain and Language 57(2): 254–79.

Harm MW (1998) A division of labor in a computational model of visual word recognition. PhD thesis. University of Southern California.

Hinton G, Shallice T (1991) Lesioning an attractor network: investigations of acquired dyslexia. Psychological Review 98: 74–95.

Landauer TK, Dumais S (1997) A solution to Plato's problem: the latent semantic analysis theory of acquisition, induction, and representation of knowledge. Psychological Review 104(2): 211–40.

Levy JP, Bullinaria JA, Patel M (1998) Explorations in the derivation of word co-occurrence statistics. South Pacific Journal of Psychology 10(1): 99–111.

McCarthy RA, Warrington EK (1988) Evidence for modality-specific meaning systems in the brain. Nature 334: 428–30.

McClelland JL (1988) Connectionist models and psychological evidence. Journal of Memory and Language 27: 107–23.

McClelland JL, Elman JL (1986) The TRACE model of speech perception. Cognitive Psychology 18: 1–86.

McClelland JL, Rumelhart DE (1981) An interactive activation model of the effect of context in perception. Psychological Review 88: 375–407.

McRae K, deSa V, Seidenberg M (1993) Modeling property intercorrelations in conceptual memory. In Polson MC, (Ed) Proceedings of the 15th Annual Conference of the Cognitive Science Society. Hillsdale, NJ: Erlbaum. pp 729–34.

McRae K, deSa VR, Seidenberg M (1997) On the nature and scope of featural representations of word meaning. Journal of Experimental Psychology: General 126(2): 99–130.

Minsky M, Papert S (1969) Perceptrons. Cambridge, MA: MIT Press.

Moss H, Tyler LK, Hodges J, Patterson K (1995) Exploring the loss of semantic memory in semantic dementia: evidence from a primed monitoring study. Neuropsychology 9(1): 16–26.

Moss HE, Tyler LK, Durrant-Peatfield M, Levy JP, Morris J (1996) Conceptual structure and category-specific deficits: drawing distinctions and identifying similarities. Second International Congress on Memory, Padova, Italy.

Patel M (1996) Using neural nets to investigate lexical analysis. In Foo N, Goebel R, (Eds) PRICAI 96: Topics in Artificial Intelligence: Proceedings of the 4th Pacific Rim International Conference on Artificial Intelligence. Berlin and Heidelberg: Springer-Verlag. pp 241–52.

Plaut D (1992) Relearning after damage in connectionist networks: implications for patient rehabilitation. In Kruschke JK, (Ed) Proceedings of the 14th Annual Conference of the Cognitive Science Society. Hillsdale, NJ: Lawrence Erlbaum Associates. pp 372–77.

Plaut D (1995) Semantic and associative priming in a distributed attractor network. Proceedings of the 17th Annual Conference of the Cognitive Science Society. Mahwah, NJ: Erlbaum. pp 37–42.

Plaut DC (1996) Relearning after damage in connectionist networks. Brain and Language 52: 25–82.

Plaut D, Shallice P (1993) Deep dyslexia: a case study of connectionist cognitive neuropsychology. Cognitive Neuropsychology 10: 377–500.

Silveri MC, Gainotti G (1988) Interaction between vision and language in category-specific semantic impairment. Cognitive Neuropsychology 5: 677–709.

Small S, Hart H, Nguyen T, Gordon B (1995) Distributed representations of semantic knowledge in the brain. Brain 118: 441–53.

Tyler LK, Moss H (1997) Functional properties of concepts: studies of normal and brain-damaged patients. Cognitive Neuropsychology 14(4): 511–45.

Warrington EK, McCarthy RA (1983) Category specific access dysphasia. Brain 106: 859–78.

Warrington EK, McCarthy RA (1987) Categories of knowledge: further fractionation and an attempted integration. Brain 110: 1273–96.

Warrington EK, Shallice T (1984) Category specific semantic impairments. Brain 107: 829–54.

Zorzi M, Perry C, Ziegler J, Coltheart M (1999) Category-specific deficits in a self-organizing model of the lexical-semantic system. In Heinke D, Humphreys GW, Olson AC, (Eds) Connectionist Models in Cognitive Neuroscience. London: Springer-Verlag.

CHAPTER 3

Putting thoughts into verbs: developmental and acquired impairments

MARIA BLACK AND SHULA CHIAT

Introduction

Linguistic meanings are extremely diverse. As the history of philosophy, linguistics and psychology shows, no single definition of meaning can encompass the wide spectrum of meanings created through human languages. In some cases, language simply wraps up bundles of perceptual and cognitive properties in a fairly straightforward one-to-one relation between concepts and the forms that express them. In most cases, however, the relation is more complex. Individual forms (words) and their combinations (phrases and sentences) rework the conceptual material to create new patterns that cut across pre-existing concepts, or reassemble old concepts into different meanings.

Although some of the basic stuff of what we call 'meaning' is already there, most meanings are created in a complex interaction of conceptual processing and linguistic systems. The meanings of verbs and other linguistic items that express relational meanings are good examples of such complex interactions. For instance, our perceptual and kinaesthetic experience can provide us with the basic concepts expressed by verbs of motion like *walk, stroll, run, hop* but the aspects of the movement we select depend on the language we use to talk about that motion – not all languages express the same manners of motion as English does. Similarly, our spatial experiences may provide us with concepts of motion in particular directions but which motions and which directions are packaged together into a single verb again depends on the language. Relative to other languages, English has a wide range of verbs expressing motion and manner but a much more restricted set of verbs like *rise* and *fall* where motion and direction are packaged together into a single verb (Naigles, Eisenberg, Kako et al., 1998; Slobin, 1996).

Some aspects of meaning can be extracted only from our linguistic experience. Verbs like *come* and *go* can be said to express pure motion or orientation. But only our experience with language, as speakers, addressees and observers of other people's linguistic interactions, can make us understand that *come* and *go* express motion or orientation towards or away from the speaker. Without language and discourse we would have no concept of 'the speaker'.

Cross-linguistic, psycholinguistic and developmental research has increasingly provided evidence that language does not simply reflect our concepts but stretches, reshapes and expands our conceptual range, exercising a powerful pull on conceptual development. Language can move children on from more 'concrete, situated and contextually embedded' comparisons to the identification of more general and abstract patterns (Gentner and Medina, 1998). As Gentner and Rattermann say (1991, cited in Gentner and Medina, 1998) 'a word can function as a promissory note signalling subtle commonalities that the child does not yet perceive.'

The role language plays in directing attention to selected aspects of experience, 'subtle commonalities' and cross-situational patterns is likely to continue into adulthood. Several theorists, from different perspectives and for different reasons, have argued that language acts as part of our system of 'selective attention' constraining what we attend to when we talk, write or sign (Gumperz and Levinson, 1996; Jackendoff, 1997; Naigles et al., 1998; Slobin, 1996; Tomlin, 1997).

The effect of language on attention is not total or totally constraining: we can conceive and direct our attention to aspects of experience different from those embodied in our language. Indeed, several attentional systems may compete when we are trying to sift through the mass of information from which we select a 'message'. But the language(s) we speak will push us towards attending more closely to some aspects of a situation we talk about (Slobin, 1996). Meyer, Sleiderink and Levelt (1998) provide evidence that the time taken to view objects in pictures before verbal description 'depended systematically on the time needed to retrieve the phonological form of the object names'. Dipper (1999) argues that effects of language can be detected at early stages of what Slobin calls 'thinking for speaking' in tasks where the encoding of a situation (an event or state) and its participants is required. It seems that we don't simply construct a message and then select the language to convey it in. Language plays a role in the selection and shaping of the message itself.

These are the central themes of this chapter: first, that linguistic meanings cannot be reduced to pre-existing conceptual packages and that meanings are created in the interaction between concepts and linguistic form. We need, therefore, to define more precisely and take into account how particular languages carve up the conceptual space and the specific properties of the forms employed in doing so. In analysing the development and impairment of verb meanings and phrasal combinations that express situations, we have to take into account conceptual, semantic and form-related properties. Unless we do so, we shall not be able to overcome 'the difficulty of interpreting the mosaic patterns of aphasic performance using two-dimensional serial models' (Berndt, Haendiges, Mitchum et al., 1997b).

Secondly, we need to analyse and model the specific meaning-form interactions that take place in particular types of tasks. Although the same types of representations may be involved in comprehension and production, impairment is likely to have different consequences for 'thinking for speaking' as opposed to 'thinking for listening'.

The chapter starts with the shaping of meaning in normal development, and the repercussions of developmental language impairment on meaning, with a specific focus on verb and sentence meaning. We then consider verb and sentence meanings in relation to acquired aphasia in adults.

Normal development: the logical case

In acquiring their language, it is clear that children must make connections between linguistic forms and the scenes in which they meet these. The meanings that the child attaches to linguistic forms must derive from the sense she has made or is making of the world around her. However, the child's task is not simply a matter of mapping the forms she hears on to pre-existing and independently established notions as is commonly assumed. This is because words and structures are not in a simple correspondence with notions about the world. If the child treated linguistic forms as labels for independently established concepts, and approached language acquisition by looking for linguistic forms to attach to those concepts, she could not possibly attain the lexical and sentential semantics of her particular language.

To illustrate the point, we start with the case of nouns naming concrete objects. The correspondence between linguistic forms and perceptual categories is at its tightest in this case, yet it is still not watertight. Take the most overt word learning situation, where the child is introduced to a word by ostension: the adult says *cup* while pointing to a cup. Assume the child's understanding of the world leads her to focus on the whole object, rather than a part or property of that object, an assumption for which there is considerable evidence (see, for example, Clark, 1993). Assume that the child maps the form /kʌp/ on to the whole object to which her attention is directed. This still does not guarantee that she has established the semantics of *cup*. Does *cup* refer to any vessel you drink out of? A vessel of a particular shape? Anything with a handle on it? No observation about the world can on its own distinguish between these possibilities. Only by encountering *the same phonological form* in the context of different exemplars of cups, and encountering *different phonological forms* in the context of things that are similar to cups but not cups, can the child establish the semantic boundaries of *cup*.

When we turn to words encoding properties, relations, states and events, even where these are of a sensori-motor nature, the word–world correspondence is markedly looser. Take the meanings of verbs such as *play, eat, fall, come, go, take, give, put*. These do not correspond to discrete aspects of scenes and cannot be pointed out. The looseness of the relationship between verb and scene is well demonstrated in a study by Gleitman and Gillette (1995). In this study, adult subjects were shown a silent video of mothers playing with their infants. They were told that a beep would sound whenever the mother used a target word, and their task was to guess that word. Where the target was a noun, they guessed correctly 50% of the time on first exposure, and they improved on this with further exposures. When the target was a verb, on the other hand, they identified that verb correctly less than 15% of the time. Clearly, for these adult subjects, the pragmatic context was a strong cue in identifying the reference of nouns but not verbs.

The situation in which these adults find themselves mimics in some crucial respects the situation of the language-acquiring child. She too must identify the reference of unknown verbs which she encounters in the course of pragmatic interactions. To get anywhere near their semantics, the child must surely be adept at focusing on a salient aspect of the scenes in which verbs are heard and one which is the focus of the speaker's attention at the time of uttering the word (Chiat, 2000; Tomasello, 1995). But however sophisticated the child's interpretation of scenes and speaker focus, it is still not enough to identify the precise semantics of these words. It is not enough, for example, to establish whether *put* refers to an event or a state or a location, or exactly what event, state or location. Only by encountering the phonological form /pʊt/ in many scenes can the child discover what distinguishes *put* from *move, get dressed, on, off*, and so on.

To the English speaker who has acquired *put*, it may seem that the verb maps on to a clearly observable and naturally categorized event, and that the child's task is a straightforward one. Comparison with a language such as Korean puts paid to such illusions. In Korean, events expressed by the single verb *put* in English are expressed by different verbs depending on the tightness of fit between the two objects involved. Korean, on the other hand, does not worry about the precise direction of movement which would be indicated in English by particles such as *in* and *on*. So the Korean child must acquire one verb for the events shown in Figures 1 and 2 as (b) and (d), which English would convey in different ways: *putting* a cassette *in* a case and *putting* a lid *on* a container. And she must acquire two separate verbs for the events shown in Figures 1 and 2 as (a) and (b), which English would represent in the same way: *putting* an apple *in* a bowl and *putting* a cassette *in* a case (Bowerman, 1996). Presumably children

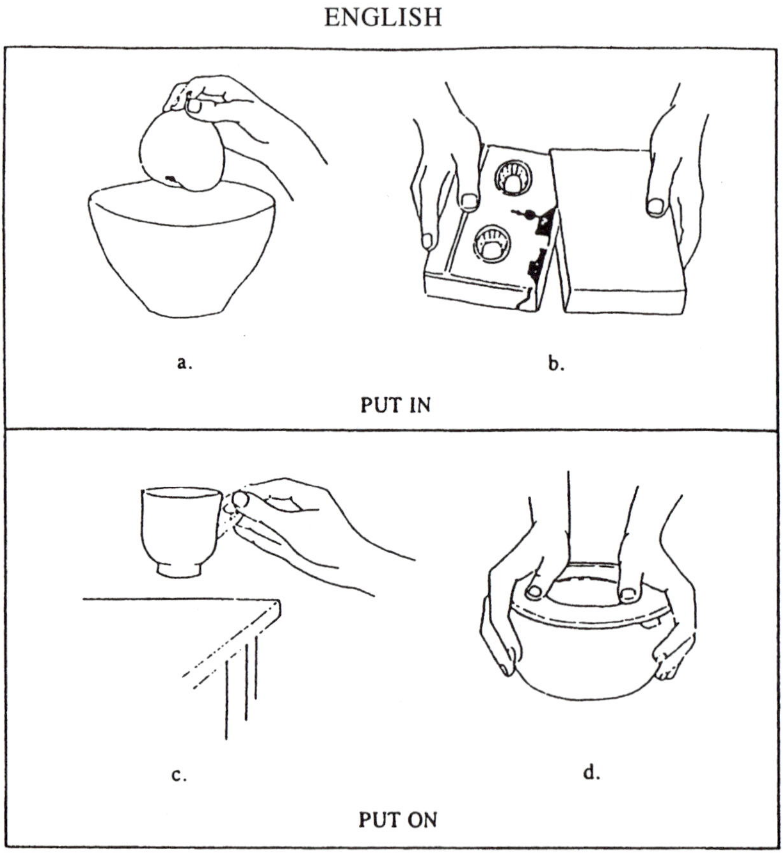

ENGLISH

From Gumperz JJ, Levinson SC (Eds) (1996) Rethinking Linguistic Relativity. Cambridge: Cambridge University Press. Reprinted by permission of Cambridge University Press.

Figure 1. Semantic classification of four actions in English.

KOREAN

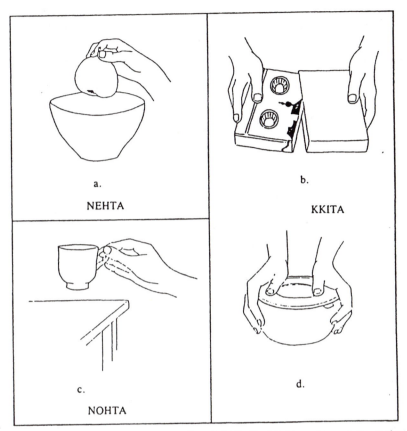

a.

NEHTA

b.

KKITA

c.

NOHTA

d.

From Gumperz JJ, Levinson SC (Eds) (1996) Rethinking Linguistic Relativity. Cambridge: Cambridge University Press. Reprinted by permission of Cambridge University Press.

Figure 2. Semantic classification of four actions in Korean.

start off with an equal capacity to acquire the semantics of movement terms in Korean and English. The semantic differences between these movement terms cannot be demonstrated or made transparent in the scene itself. Only the constant linguistic representation – the word phonology observed in different scenes – can cue the child to its meaning.

Word-size phonology, though, is not always sufficient to cue semantics. Where words encode *meaning relations*, it is not always possible to retrieve their relational meaning fully by finding correspondences between word and world. Fisher, Hall, Rakowitz et al., (1994), and Gleitman and Gillette (1995) have argued cogently that the acquisition of *verb meanings* requires sentence-to-world rather than word-to-world mappings. Verbs refer to events which, even in the most everyday cases, typically involve complex relations between entities. Take a simple event such as a change of possession. Perceptually, this involves one individual with an object moving their hand and another individual moving their hand to end up with that object. This event could be seen from the perspective of either individual. When we refer to the event, we must select one or other perspective, these being differentiated in the verbs *give* and *take*. We have no single verb that refers to the entire event, regardless of perspective, or incorporating both perspectives. When children hear these verbs, the scene will typically allow interpretation from either perspective. How does the child know which perspective the verb expresses? The focus in the scene at that moment in time may provide a cue: the child may notice that the speaker is focused on the source of the transfer and infer that *give* takes the perspective of the source. A more reliable cue, however, is the syntactic position of the verb's arguments. Noticing which argument – source or goal – occupies the subject position will indicate the verb's perspective on the event.

A similar case has been made for events involving the movement of one entity in relation to a second entity that changes state as a result, for example pouring juice which fills a cup. When hearing a verb in the context of such events, the child must discover whether that verb focuses on the movement (*pour*) or the result (*fill*). A crucial cue is the syntactic position of the entity that moves and the entity that changes state. The direct object picks out the more focused entity; the less focused entity may occur in a prepositional phrase. Noticing which entities are included, and where they occur, the child could distinguish the perspective taken by the verb:

- The woman is pouring juice (into the cup) – focus on moved object.
- The woman is filling the cup (with juice) – focus on affected object.
- The woman is putting the cloth on the table – focus on moved object.
- The woman is covering the table with the cloth – focus on affected object.

Again, we find examples of cross-linguistic variation in the details of event perspective. Different languages, for example, may prefer one or other perspective on everyday psychological states. While English goes for *like* and *need*, Spanish and Italian go for *please* and *lack*. Children cannot know in advance which perspective their language takes on these states.

Only the configuration of stimulus and experiencer arguments can reveal this. The use of syntactic configurations to determine the focus of the verb has come to be known as 'syntactic bootstrapping' (Fisher et al.,1994).

If the child is to carry out syntactic bootstrapping, she must register the phonological forms and sequence of at least the verb and the relevant argument(s). This implies that the acquisition of a crucial aspect of verb meaning – event perspective – depends on more than single word phonology and its relation to the scene.

Normal development: empirical evidence

Children's earliest utterances convey meanings which are linguistically shaped. The clearest empirical evidence lies in fine-grained comparison between the semantics of early words in children acquiring different languages. On the one hand, children in different linguistic environments have been noted to express very similar meanings. At the one-to-two word utterance stage, children typically use 'basic-level' terms for objects and people (Clark,1993); they use terms and word combinations which refer to states and changes of state, locations and changes of location, possession (Bloom, 1970; Braine, 1976; Brown, 1973). But when we look at the precise meanings and forms by which these broader meanings are conveyed, children show the influence of their particular language.

English-speaking children show a preponderance of nouns, with verbs and other predicate terms forming a small proportion of their vocabulary at this stage (Gentner, 1982; Nelson, 1973). They have also been found to use nouns productively before they do so with verbs. In a study by Tomasello, Akhtar, Dodson et al., (1997), 22-month-old children who were taught novel nouns and verbs produced novel combinations with the nouns (for example *Wug gone* or *More wug*) but not with the verbs.

Compare the profile of one-to-two-word-stage Korean. In a study of 10 children aged 1;2–1;10, Choi (1997) found similar proportions of nouns and verbs in their early vocabularies: nouns 44%, verbs 31%. For an equivalent group of English-speaking children, the proportions were nouns 65%, verbs 6%. Choi attributes this difference in acquisition to differences in phonological, syntactic and pragmatic characteristics of verbs in the input to English- and Korean-speaking children. In Korean, verbs occur clause-finally and are more likely to occur in isolation (without arguments) than in English. Furthermore, Korean mothers talking to children were found to use more action verbs than English mothers, who used more object nouns than their Korean counterparts.

The comparison of language acquisition in Korean and English is salutary. It demonstrates clearly that observable events and linguistic forms are not in a one-to-one relationship, and hence that observation of scenes is not sufficient to determine the meaning of verb forms. It further demonstrates that, from the earliest stages of language production, meaning is shaped by the forms and structures of the language. According to Choi,

> The semantic categories of the youngest age group in each language are significantly more similar to those of the adult group of the corresponding language than to same-age group learning the other language. (Choi, 1997: 86–7)

This understanding of what is involved in learning to convey events has important implications for possible sources of impairment in the acquisition of verbs and verb structure.

Implications for developmental impairments

If the source of linguistic meaning is the sense the child makes of the world, an infant who makes limited or different sense of the world will clearly have problems with linguistic meaning. The ways in which she perceives objects, people, their characteristics and relations, including her perception of other people's perception of these, will be the material onto which she maps the linguistic forms she encounters. The extent to which the child matches the meanings of her language will depend on the extent to which she shares others' perception and interpretation of the world. If many aspects of her perception and interpretation are intact, she could succeed in establishing many aspects of word and sentence meaning and use these correctly in many contexts. Limitations in her meanings would become apparent only in contexts that entail aspects of perception or interpretation which she lacks. Suppose a child interprets visual and motor experiences in the same way as other people and recognizes others' visuo-motor perspectives, but has limited or no understanding of emotional or mental experience. In this case, meanings rooted in the visuo-motor domain may be intact. The child may refer to physical objects and events quite appropriately. Meanings rooted in emotional or mental experience, on the other hand, will be either missing, or inappropriately mapped on to visual or motor categories associated with them. We might expect the child not to use emotional or mental terms, or to use them only in contexts where they have visible or tangible effects (Chiat, 2000).

Logically, deficits in a child's interpretation of the world must affect the meanings that the child attaches to forms or structures which rest on that interpretation. The logical consequences of deficits in linguistic form are less immediately obvious, but flow from our analysis of the way that linguistic form shapes meaning.

A child who has difficulties processing linguistic forms and structures may have no difficulty interpreting the world: she sets out with the same sense of objects, people, their characteristics and relations as other children. However, we have seen how, from the earliest stages, the child's encounter with particular forms across different scenes determines which aspects of those scenes she notices, and the meanings that she establishes. If the child has difficulty segmenting phonological chunks and holding them across contexts, she will have difficulty discovering the semantic scope of words. The extent of this difficulty will depend in part on the extent of her difficulties with phonology. The more limited and unstable her phonological representations, the less these will cue her to semantic constancy and difference across contexts. The effects on her semantic representations will depend on properties of those semantic representations and the forms by which they are expressed, which may make them more or less vulnerable to phonological weakness, as outlined in the following predictions.

- The closer a target semantic representation is to a pre-linguistic perceptually-based concept, the easier it will be to establish. Concrete nouns therefore have the greatest advantage.
- Conversely, the more a semantic representation depends on language, the more dependent it is on phonological representation, and the less accessible it will be to the child. We should therefore expect greater difficulty with verbs, whose relation to the observable world is less direct.
- Where the establishment of semantic representations depends on their phonological representation, the relative difficulty of their phonology will be a further factor in acquisition. The more phonologically challenging they are, the more vulnerable they will be. Meanings expressed by stressed words or stressed syllables, and even unstressed syllables that follow stress, will be more accessible than unstressed syllables that precede stress (Chiat, 2000; Slobin, 1973). For example, aspects of meaning expressed in verbs should be more accessible than those expressed in unstressed prepositions.
- The more dependent semantic representations are on sentence-to-world mapping, as opposed to word-to-world mapping, the more phonology and syntactic relations must be processed, and the more challenging they will be. Hence, aspects of an event that can be identified from observation of the event, for example, manner of movement, or emotional state, should be more accessible than aspects that depend on organization of arguments in relation to the verb, such as perspective on movement or on emotional state. Examples of such meanings

are the perspective differences between verbs such as *give/take, buy/sell, fill/pour, amuse/enjoy.*

How do these predictions match up with the evidence?

Evidence from developmental impairments

It is well established that developmental language impairments affect some aspects of language more than others. This becomes apparent when language-impaired children are matched with normally developing children on some linguistic measure, such as vocabulary age or MLU, and are found to diverge, to varying degrees, on other linguistic measures. The relative difficulty of different aspects of language appears to fit our predictions. For example, discussing language-impaired children who are beginning to produce multi-word utterances, Leonard observes that:

> Verbs, in particular, begin to show deficiencies that seem to go beyond the general lag in these children's lexical abilities. (1998: 44)

This is illustrated by studies of verb use in spontaneous samples produced by language-impaired children. Watkins, Rice and Moltz (1993) calculated type token ratios (TTRs) for a group of 14 language-impaired children and groups of age-matched and language-matched controls. The language-impaired subjects showed lower TTRs for *verbs* than the controls, but their *overall* TTRs did not differ. This means that the language-impaired children used a less diverse range of verbs than their normally developing counterparts.

In an analysis of verb use by three language-impaired children aged between 3;8 and 4;8, Rice and Bode (1993) observed a number of errors. These children sometimes omitted a verb, for example:

I my flowers back	for	I want my flowers back
Let me that	for	Let me do that.

They also produced verbs that were inappropriate for the semantic context. In some cases, the substitution was an over-general verb:

You *get* in that guy and it'll work

where *push* would have been appropriate;

I'm *doing* two balloons

where *use, bounce, juggle, play with* would have been appropriate. In other cases, the substitution was semantically related to the target:

Birds live to California   for   Birds go to California
(fixed location instead of change of location);

Spray this   for   Sprinkle this
(wrong manner of movement).

What is particularly surprising about the substitution and omission of verbs is that very often the child produced the missing verb correctly in other contexts. A child who had substituted an over-general verb for *catch*, *push*, *play*, and *throw* had at some point used each of these verbs. Another child who used *read* correctly 24 times and *write* correctly 11 times once used *read* for *write* and once used *write* for *draw*. The majority of verb omissions occurred in contexts calling for precisely those verbs that were used with high frequency in other contexts.

These findings were replicated in an in-depth single case study of Travis, a 6-year-old language-impaired child (Chiat, 2000; Evelyn, 1996). In this study, event descriptions were elicited by acting out 127 events and asking Travis to say what had happened. His event descriptions were compared with those proffered by three younger, vocabulary-matched subjects. These normally developing 4-year-olds made few errors in verb use: omission of verbs or their arguments was virtually non-existent, and only a handful of substitutions occurred. In contrast, Travis omitted verbs in 22 of his event descriptions, for example:

For emptying a bottle: Thing out
For rocking arms: Wobbly jelly.

He also made unusual substitutions:

For pushing a pram: Drive [ə] baby chair.

Like the subjects in the Rice and Bode study, almost all omissions occurred in contexts calling for a verb which Travis successfully used in other contexts. The verb *tip* which he used in his description of emptying a jar ('Tip in there') would have served perfectly well for the emptying of a bottle, for which his description was verbless ('Thing out'). He used the verb *rock* for rocking side to side ('Rocking'), but did not produce a verb for rocking arms ('Wobbly jelly').

Travis' production of verbs and verb structure was further investigated in a set of picture description and repetition tasks with matched targets. In the picture description task, he was shown a set of pictures and asked to make a sentence using a particular verb, for example *chase, put, give, buy, take, sell*. As in the event description task, his score was well below that of the controls, and he made errors of a sort that never occurred in the controls' responses. As well as omissions, he used multiple verbs to convey certain events, for example:

(Picture shows sheep selling pear to pig; the verb *sell* is supplied)
Travis: Pig want – want pear in basket – sheep give it pig – pig want pear – um basket and sheep and he give it and lot – lot of 5p.

(Picture shows panda buying pear from monkey; the verb *buy* is supplied)
Travis: Monkey – panda want a pear – monkey want money.

These responses included relevant aspects of the event, but failed to integrate these into a single verb.

In repetition without pictures, Travis was asked to repeat the set of sentences that were the targets in the picture description task. Here, his score plunged even further. While the controls were close to ceiling (scores ranging from 89% to 98%), Travis scored 20%. His responses to repetition were distinguished by omissions and substitution with unintelligible 'fillers', for example:

Target: The pig chases the sheep
Travis: [ə] pig [ə] sheep.

Interestingly, in repetition *with pictures*, where he viewed the pictures corresponding to the sentences, his verb-argument structures were quantitatively and qualitatively similar to his picture descriptions.

In summary, Travis' pattern of performance showed omissions and substitutions of verbs and arguments which almost never occurred in the responses of the younger language-matched controls. These omissions and substitutions were more extreme where the stimuli were purely linguistic (repetition without pictures) than where the stimuli included pictures (picture description and repetition with pictures).

Collectively, the findings of these studies indicate particular problems with verbs and verb structure. The nature of these difficulties presents a conundrum. On the one hand, there is evidence that these children understand relevant aspects of events for which they fail to produce full verbs (their use of the required verb in other contexts, Travis's use of multiple verb substitutions). There is also evidence that they have semantic, phonological and syntactic representations required to map these events (their use of the correct verb and structure in some contexts). What, then, leads to the limitations, omissions and substitutions we have observed? According to Evelyn (1996) and Chiat (2000), weaknesses in mapping events on to verb structure are the ultimate product of weak phonological processing and representations (see the previous section where the role of phonology in acquiring verbs is discussed).

To evaluate this broad claim, and other possible explanations for the inconsistencies we have observed, we need to probe these children's verb processing further. Current evidence is too limited to determine what makes verbs more or less accessible in output. We also have little evidence of what these children know about verbs in input. Our discussion of normal development provides clear pointers towards questions we might usefully explore. Are there differences between the events for which a verb is used successfully, and those for which it is omitted or substituted? Are verbs of certain semantic types more accessible than others? Are any such differences echoed in the child's comprehension of verbs: do they show understanding of some aspects of verb meaning or some categories of verbs, but not others? Some of these issues have been explored in relation to acquired aphasia.

Evidence from acquired impairments in adults

Acquired impairments in adults affect a fully developed system of world-to-word and world-to-sentence mappings. We must, therefore, be cautious in making predictions. It would be theoretically and empirically unwise to predict a 'hierarchy of difficulty' applicable to all types of adult aphasia and directly parallel to the developmental patterns we have discussed. Relative difficulty depends on the nature of the impairment and its specific effects on processing. We will not claim that the meaning-form mappings that are acquired later, or are developmentally most challenging, are especially vulnerable to breakdown. Nevertheless, some of the theoretical distinctions we have drawn on in relation to development are useful in interpreting different patterns of difficulty, or dissociations, in acquired aphasia.

First of all, there is considerable evidence that perceptual, concrete aspects of meaning can be affected separately from more abstract and language-dependent aspects. Many adults with aphasia have been shown to have less difficulty in producing nouns that refer to concrete, perceptually identifiable objects. For instance, three of the patients – JG, EM and LC – studied by Byng (1988) and Byng, Nickels and Black (1994) showed a significant advantage in producing nouns to describe pictures of concrete objects (e.g. the noun *iron*) than in producing phonologically identical verbs to describe pictures of related events (the verb *iron*). The same pattern of relative difficulty was found by Dipper (1999) for four of the patients in her study (LH, LS, RB, and RK) using the same materials and task.

The reverse pattern, although more rare, has also been documented. RG, the patient with acquired jargon aphasia studied by Marshall, Chiat, Robson et al. (1996), was still able to distinguish aspects of meaning dependent on linguistic perspective (e.g. *buy/sell*) and had access to thematic properties of verbs that allowed him to identify participants in an event by their role with respect to the verb. For instance, after hearing a sentence like *Aberdeen is chasing Ealing*, he could reliably pick out the Aberdeen or Ealing characters by using the information that they were either chasing or being chased. On the other hand, he was less reliable at picking out characters or objects in pictures when these were identified by ordinary common nouns rather than their role in a situation (Marshall, Black, and Byng, 1999). RG had more difficulty in accessing concrete, perceptually-based aspects of meaning and would produce semantic substitutions that involved such semantic contrasts, e.g. *swing* for *skip*; *sit* for *stand*. Marshall et al. (1996) argue that

> RG's semantic system sustained damage in the concrete, perceptual domains. As a result, he was particularly disadvantaged with words which encode most of their features in those domains . . . This brought about the reverse concreteness effect with nouns and the advantage for verbs. (258)

A similar analysis is suggested by Breedin, Saffran and Coslett (1994) for DM who on tests of semantic knowledge showed a disproportionate loss for perceptual properties of things. DM's loss of perceptual information cut across nouns and verbs, making it more plausible to think of his impairment as one affecting some types of conceptual or semantic information rather than particular classes of words.

However, the contrast between concrete, perceptually-based properties and more abstract, language-dependent ones may not be the only reason why some adults with aphasia find verbs more difficult than nouns or vice versa. Other semantic properties or features of meaning-form mappings might be at the root of such differential patterns of difficulty. The verbs in the picture naming task used by Byng (1988), Byng et al. (1994) and Dipper (1999) all express concrete actions that are quite specific and stable in their perceptual correlates. Especially for the set of verbs that express actions carried out with a particular type of instrument (e.g. *iron, hoover, mop, rake*), how the action can be carried out does not vary much from situation to situation and there is a limited range of possible participants – the actor is usually human and the entities in relation to which the action is carried out are usually inanimate and of predictable, limited types. Thus, many of the noun/verb pairs are fairly close in terms of degree of concreteness and the nature of the perceptual information involved. Nevertheless, some aphasic people still found it more difficult to access and/or produce the word form for the object than for the corresponding action. This means that even when the level of concreteness or perceptual definition is close, there is still a contrast between how we think about and name concrete things and actions (McCarthy and Warrington, 1985; Williams and Canter, 1987; Zingeser and Berndt, 1990).

The relevant contrast might have to be stated more generally as one between individual entities, concrete or otherwise, and relations between individual entities, be they actions, events or states. Indeed, a more general difference between entities and relations might be at the root of the differential patterns of impairment with nouns and verbs that have been shown in several studies of adults with acquired aphasia.

Once the relevant representations are established, relations might not always be more difficult to process than entities. What looks more likely is that they are processed differently, with different mechanisms being involved and affected by language breakdown. So we find that many patients with aphasia have greater difficulties in producing and/or comprehending verbs than nouns. More rarely, we also find the opposite pattern, with verbs being easier than nouns.

Like children with SLI, adults with verb problems omit verbs in a variety of production tasks, e.g.

ROX: the man is sack of potatoes (*carrying* omitted, picture description, McCarthy and Warrington, 1985).
JG: the iron (describing a picture of a woman ironing, Byng, 1988).
AER: Cinderella shoe (story telling, Nickels, Byng and Black, 1991).
EM: the hoover (describing a picture of a woman hoovering, Marshall, Pring and Chiat, 1998).
SS: Eyes. Chair, chair (for *looking out of the window*, in constrained production, Breedin, Saffran and Schwartz, 1998).

They may substitute semantically related verbs for the target verbs they are unable to produce, e.g.

ML: The grandmother was kissing the boy (for *hugging* in constrained elicitation, Mitchum and Berndt, 1994).
PB: The girl is hoovering the towels (for *ironing* in picture description, Marshall, Chiat and Pring, 1997).

They also produce nouns in verb positions, often using the noun for an object involved in the situation, e.g.

> ROX: the daughter was chairing (for *sitting on the chair*, McCarthy and Warrington, 1985).
> EM: The man is globing the world (cued production with noun *globe*, Marshall et al., 1998).

Different patterns of noun/verb difficulty are not typical of any particular syndrome and have been found in adults who fall within different clinical categories, with varying degrees of impairment (see Berndt, Haendiges, Mitchum et al., 1997a) and for speakers of different languages (Miceli, Silveri, Nocentini et al., 1984; Bates, Chen, Tzeng et al., 1991). In spite of 'the mosaic patterns of aphasic performance' (Berndt et al., 1997b) it is clear from recent reviews of the literature that greater difficulty with verbs cannot be explained as a symptom of a general 'syntactic deficit' (see Berndt et al., 1997a, 1997b; Bates et al., 1991; Devescovi, Bates, D'Amico et al., 1997).

What is not clear from the literature is how to interpret exactly what surfaces as a noun/verb contrast. Are meaning-related properties more important than form-related properties? Or, as we are suggesting, do we have to take into account meaning, form and their interaction?

In spite of the number of studies carried out, the types of semantic properties that have been identified and investigated are still fairly limited. Only the specific contrast between object and actions, and differences in concreteness and abstractness have been studied in any depth (but see Breedin et al., 1998).

In their conclusions to one of the most extensive and systematic studies of noun/verb differences, Berndt et al. (1997a) argue that

> . . . these results provide evidence that some selective word class differences actually reflect the influence of grammatical class (noun/verb) rather than semantic category (action/object). The two patients whose oral reading data were not subject to floor effects (FM and ML) maintained clear noun/verb differences with abstract stimulus words that were not members of the semantic categories of concrete objects and pictureable actions . . . On the basis of these results, we assume that focal brain damage can affect content words selectively as a function of their usage in the grammatical classes of noun and verb. (96)

While we would agree that noun/verb dissociations cannot be reduced to the semantic object/action distinction, it doesn't follow that semantics does not matter. When we look at the list of abstract nouns and verbs used by Berndt et al., we find that all of the abstract verbs express relations (e.g.

events or states like *deny, owe, respond, deserve*) while many of the abstract nouns express entities, albeit ones without perceptual or physical correlates (e.g. *ego, fate, democracy, miracle*). What we do not know is whether patients would continue to show a difference between nouns and verbs when both the noun and the verb express relations. Would there still be a difference for noun/verb pairs like *walk, jump, swim, kick, murder, lecture, love, dislike, hope?* Although phonologically and orthographically identical noun/verb pairs have been tested in sentence contexts (Caramazza and Hillis, 1991; Hillis and Caramazza, 1995; Rapp and Caramazza, 1998) the noun and verb have either expressed different conceptual categories (e.g. *watch*, the object versus *watch*, the relation) or mixed lists have been used with nouns and verbs like *watch* together with nouns and verbs like *walk*. To our knowledge, the two types of meaning-form mappings have not been systematically distinguished and compared in aphasia research.

If, as we would argue, the relevant distinction at the conceptual or semantic level is the one between entities and relations, there may well be gradations of difficulty within each category that could affect the meaning-form mapping. Entities that are mainly specified by their perceptual properties (concrete objects) may be easier than those that have more abstract and general properties (abstract entities). Relations that have perceptual correlates, apply to specific types of entities, and vary little from context to context, may be easier than relations with less or no perceptual specification and which are more general in their application to types of entities and situations. For instance, the event expressed by the English verb *eat* may be easier than the event expressed by the verb *open* because, although they both have perceptual correlates, the range of situations that can be labelled by the verb *open* is wider than the range picked out by the verb *eat*. As long as a certain result is brought about, how and what we open is irrelevant in English. In another language, however, there may be different verbs for opening depending on the type of action involved and what is being opened. Relative difficulty, therefore, will be partly conceptual and partly semantic – that is, language-specific. How different languages package conceptual material should be taken into account when we interpret the performance of aphasic people within and across languages.

Nevertheless, as we have already argued in relation to development, the properties of the form are also important – not only its frequency but also its syntactic and phonological characteristics. Where a form can occur in a sentence, what it can combine with, what prosodic patterns it has, all could make a difference. For instance, in comparison to nouns, disyllabic English verbs tend to have the less frequent prosodic pattern with stress on the second syllable, both as a set and in comparison to their related nouns (e.g. 'record/re'cord; 'rebel/re'bel; 'transport/tran'sport). Such form-related properties may have more or less of an effect depending on the type of task and the type of impairment involved – form or meaning may tip the processing balance in any one case. The most robust and stable effects may be obtained where form and meaning converge as in, for instance, the abstract noun and verb comparisons in the study by Berndt et al.(1997a). In that condition, all the verbs express relations and 7 out of 12 verbs have stress on the second syllable, while only about half of the nouns express relations and only 3 out of 12 nouns have stress on the second syllable (a convergence of semantic, syntactic and prosodic properties).

Syntactic category, or word class, is a form-related property that may conflict with meaning. In this respect, we would agree with those researchers who have argued for a form-related representation of syntactic properties, separate from meaning (see Caramazza and Miozzo, 1997; Rapp and Caramazza, 1997). Although certain types of concepts (e.g. concrete objects) are regularly mapped on to certain types of syntactic categories (nouns), in many other cases both in individual languages and cross-linguistically, meaning and syntactic category do not go hand in hand. As we have already seen, some actions, processes and states (relations) can be nouns or verbs. It is precisely because meaning and form are distinct that language allows us the flexibility to talk about relations as if they were 'things'. Compare, for instance, the nouns *walk* and *sleep* with their verb counterparts in the following sentences:

We are going to have a walk/sleep (noun)
We are going to walk/sleep (verb).

In the first sentence, we can talk about an action, presenting it as 'a participant' in a situation by using the noun, which allows us to combine it with devices like determiners. Because of the combination of noun form and determiner, we can present the action as a more clearly individuated conceptual unit with more definite boundaries – temporal boundaries rather than spatial as in the case of concrete objects. Thus, with the noun, we give the impression that we are planning to walk or sleep for a shorter time. When using the verb, on the other hand, we are simply saying that we are planning to engage in an activity that might go on for an indefinite period of time (see Frawley, 1992). The properties of the form bias us to see 'things' when we are really talking about actions.

Making a scene: verb meaning and sentence processing

We have seen that processing the meaning of words, especially of verbs, is not an all-or-none affair. Aspects of meaning may be dissociated: it is possible to retain perceptually-based aspects of meaning and lose access to more abstract, language-dependent features. Or vice versa, as in the cases of RG and DM mentioned in the previous section. Although investigations of verb meaning dissociations in aphasia are still limited, there is a common thread through many of the studies of sentence processing impairments. Loss of, or unreliable access to, verb information is linked to problems in comprehending and/or producing sentences (Berndt et al., 1997b; Byng, 1988; Byng and Black, 1989; Haendiges et al., 1996; Jones, 1984; Marshall et al., 1993; Marshall et al., 1997; Mitchum et al., 1993; Nickels et al., 1991; Schwartz et al., 1985; Schwartz et al., 1994). While there are differences in emphasis in these studies, most of them highlight a correlation between problems in accessing verb-specific thematic and perspective information, and problems in comprehending reversible SVO sentences and producing combinations of verbs and their argument phrases (see, in particular, Byng and Black, 1989; Marshall et al., 1999). For instance, Nickels et al. say that AER, one of the patients in their study,

> . . . has a deficit in the ability to access specific verb semantics . . . including information concerning thematic roles and their realization in sentence form. (1991: 180)

PB, the patient studied by Marshall et al.,

> retained information about verbs' core meanings, but not about their thematic properties . . . he was able to differentiate eat and drink . . . but not give and take. (1997: 873)

Berndt et al. conclude that

> verb retrieval problems significantly correlated with other purely structural aspects of sentence production that occur in agrammatic and other types of patients . . . The significant correlations indicate that patients who were poor at producing verbs to name actions produced fewer sentences, and simpler sentences, than did patients who were better at verb production. (1997b:128)

Given the considerable variations in specific individual patterns and in the types of verbs employed in different studies, we have to be extremely cautious in drawing general conclusions. Nevertheless, a number of trends seem worth highlighting.

First of all, it seems more likely that access to aspects of verb meaning has been impaired, or slowed down, rather than the representations themselves, since individual performance can fluctuate considerably on the same task or is affected by the nature of the task (Black et al., 1991; Cupples and Inglis, 1993 ; Friederici and Frazier, 1992). For some patients, the picture-sentence matching format, especially when multiple pictures or video scenes are presented together, creates the most acute problems. For instance, EM, one of the patients studied by Byng et al. (1994), was significantly better at comprehending sentences in a semantic anomaly judgement than in a picture matching task with similar SVO sentences. An equivalent pattern of results was obtained by Cupples and Inglis (1993).

In sentence-picture matching tasks, the nature of the verb and of the visually presented scene can make a significant difference to performance. Like Jones (1984), Haendiges et al. (1996) find that in matching reversible SVO sentences to pictures, '. . . the most consistent errors were with directional motion verbs (pull, chase, and follow).' Black et al. (1991) and Cupples and Inglis (1993) found that SVO sentences with psychological state verbs such as *admire* and *delight* were consistently more difficult to match correctly to pictures than SVO sentences with action verbs. Since the action/state effect was true of non-aphasic controls as well, Black et al. claim that the increased error rates are not due to problems with the verb per se or with some aspects of sentence processing, but arise in the construction of representations that 'mediate the translation between language and pictures' (1993: 79).

What could scenes of chasing and following have in common with scenes of admiring and delighting? Building on the analysis of Black et al. (1991), we would suggest that in all these scenes participants are not so obviously contrasted in terms of their visual and conceptual characteristics. There are fewer cues to distinguish the participant who is more 'agentive' or 'the anchoring point' from whose perspective the scene should be understood and compared with the sentence. Compare a scene of chasing or following with one of photographing or washing. Although the way the scene is depicted may make a difference, when X chases Y, both X and Y are usually moving, both are doing something – hence the notorious difficulties in analysing the thematic roles of these kinds of verbs (see, for instance, Jackendoff, 1990). The same scene could equally be described as Y running away from X. With photographing, on the other hand, there will be several converging cues to mark out one of the participants as more 'agentive', 'more causally weighted' (Black et al., 1991) and the more obvious 'anchoring point' for interpreting the scene. A linguistic description of the scene from the point of view of the person being photographed would require the passive – Y is (being) photographed by X – or a construction with *get* or *have* – X got/had his picture taken.

A similar argument can be made for the difficulty of state scenes, psychological or otherwise – hence the problems in thematic analysis for some of these verbs and the considerable cross-linguistic variation in how verbs encode psychological states (see the second section of this chapter, page 54). Note that it is not just the conceptual representation of the scene itself or just the perspective of the verb and the sentence that create the difficulties. It is in the interaction of the two, in 'the thinking for listening' that the problems arise. For aphasic people who may precisely have problems in processing the perspective of verbs and sentences, such combinations of pictured scene and verb type could be a processing double whammy.

As Haendiges et al. say, further 'systematic manipulation of the nature of the verbs used in sentences is clearly needed' (1996: 297). However, some preliminary evidence that perspective-related aspects of meaning of verbs are difficult for people with acquired aphasia is already available in the studies we have mentioned in this section (see also Breedin et al., 1998). Dipper (1999) shows that perspective-related problems can occur in comprehension even when the person can process most other aspects of verb and sentence meaning. LH, one of the participants in Dipper's study, performed well on several word and sentence comprehension tasks. She made errors only when, after seeing a video scene, she was asked to select the most appropriate verb from pairs expressing different perspectives on the same event.

While we would certainly not claim that all comprehension problems with verbs and sentences can be explained in these terms, we can give a new interpretative twist to some old data with this analysis. Effects of 'saliency' related to differential size, animacy or 'potency' have been claimed since the start of investigations into reversible sentence comprehension (Schwartz et al., 1980). Those are the kinds of factors that tend to make one participant more 'agentive' and more likely to be the 'anchoring point' of the description, taking up, for instance, the subject position in an English sentence (Sridhar, 1988; Frawley, 1992). Non-reversible sentences, which have been consistently claimed not to present problems for people with aphasia in picture-sentence matching, are at one extreme of the perspective problem continuum: the very nature of the scene ensures that the participants are presented in asymmetrical roles. Confronted with a standard depiction of eating, we could undoubtedly describe it from the point of view of the sandwich (e.g. the sandwich slipped down X's throat; the sandwich went into X's mouth) but we do not have a pair of verbs that present a different perspective on the very same event in these cases. The only other alternative would be to use a construction like the passive (the sandwich was eaten by X), which is far less frequent and subject to considerable semantic and pragmatic constraints (Black et al., 1991). At the other extreme are scenes in which an event includes two active participants, like transactions between two people.

Why should perspective, which has not figured much in the aphasia literature, make such a difference? Perspective taking is a feature of many cognitive domains and, as we illustrated in the second section, is fundamental to language. Perspective taking is therefore intrinsic to thinking for listening and thinking for speaking, as many psycholinguists have pointed out (Jackendoff, 1983, 1997; Langacker, 1997; Levelt, 1996; Pinker, 1989; Slobin, 1996). As Levelt, Roelofs and Meyer say:

> Perspective taking is not just a peculiar aspect of spatial description; rather, it is a general property of all referring. It is even an essential component in tasks as simple as picture naming. Should the object be referred to as an animal, a horse or a mare? (1999: 8–9)

Jörg and Hörmann (1978), who found significant effects of different noun labels on unimpaired picture recognition, conclude that

> . . . the choice of one or other term by the speaker . . . is not guided solely by his tendency to refer unambiguously to the object he means . . . but also by the speaker's intention to emphasize, for the hearer, how 'wide' or 'narrow' he should code what he is going to process cognitively . . . The speaker provides, by choosing between several labels . . . subtle hints as to how he wants the hearer to comprehend the situation. (1978: 453–54)

Thus, language acts as an attention-guiding device, a 'zoom lens' that focuses us on different aspects of an object both as children developing language and as adults.

As we have already argued, the attentional effects of language are bound to be stronger where perceptual systems leave us most free to choose – for instance, how we relate individual entities in a scene, what aspects of the scene we focus on and which perspective we adopt. By providing a network of relational terms and a set of basic syntactic and prosodic structures in which these terms can occur, language provides us with 'filters' or basic 'schemas' to reshape in our minds what the perceptual and cognitive systems have brought to our attention. As Slobin says:

> Each native language has trained its speakers to pay different kinds of attention to events and experiences when talking about them. (1996: 89)

If English had a single, common verb for what the sandwich does in an eating scene, English speakers might be more inclined to take the sandwich's perspective. After all, a bilingual speaker of, say, English and Italian has no difficulty in entertaining and switching between different perspectives on a feeling and its experiencer since each language makes available different linguistic means to do so.

What happens when our automatic access to the language-dependent 'scene schemas', implicit in the meaning of verbs and verb-argument combinations, is impaired? We have already hinted at what the consequences for comprehension might be. At least, in comprehension tasks, people can use the phonological or orthographic form of the verb to a greater or lesser extent; the different verbs provided may allow the person to get enough information to form a partial representation of the scene which can then be used to guide their conceptualization of the picture, although problems might arise with particular aspects of meaning or when there is a conflict between what the aphasic person manages to construct from the language input and the picture – for instance, when the sentence presents the same scene as the picture but with the participant roles reversed (Cupples and Inglis, 1993).

The consequences for production, however, are likely to be more drastic. It is not surprising, therefore, to find that even for aphasic people who have reasonable access to verbs and their associated syntactic and prosodic frames in input, production of verbs and even minimal combinations of relational terms and their arguments can be extremely hard (Marshall et al., 1998; Dipper, 1999). In their review of the literature on verb and sentence processing problems, Berndt et al. acknowledge that there is an intriguing discrepancy between input and output performance:

> It may be that an impairment to lemma representations, that is of sufficient magnitude to undermine the retrieval of a specific entry for production, does not necessarily abolish semantic information. (1997b: 98)

We would argue that such a discrepancy reflects a normal difference in how linguistic meanings are activated in input and output. Language impairment exaggerates the discrepancy. In input, activation is driven by the form one hears or sees. The form sets the process in motion. Aspects of the process may be more or less impaired or slowed down in aphasia, but there is at least enough of a trigger to get the process going. In production, on the other hand, there may be a spiral of impairment. If the network of words and constructions of a language shapes certain aspects of our 'messages', especially with regard to situations involving relations between several entities, then we might not be able to construct a specification of the message that is sufficiently detailed to trigger information to all the required aspects of the linguistic system so that an appropriate phrase or sentence can be produced.

If our interpretation is correct, then we would expect that constraining the attentional processes and selections that have to be made at the message level may have an effect on the language produced – an idea germane to the well established clinical assumption that, for some patients, the more you constrain and structure what they are trying to communicate, the most successful the communication.

When we consider some of the verb and 'mapping' therapies that have been employed with some success with aphasic adults we find that many of them, in different ways, are exercises in thinking for speaking. For instance, Jones (1986) says that her therapy with BB aimed to clarify 'what was entailed in the concept of a particular verb.' Nickels, Byng and Black were trying to '. . . make explicit to AER the relationship between the roles of the participants in an event and the relative position in the sentence of the NPs expressing those participants' (1991: 184). Marshall et al. (1993) were working '. . . to identify the roles played by the participants in events and to improve her focus on the nature of the action or verb.' By explicitly focusing on different aspects of a scene and their translations into language, and, conversely, by providing a variety of instances of scenes all labelled by the same verb and sentence structure, some of these therapies may precisely have an effect on thinking for speaking. By taking into account the complex interaction between concepts, meanings and linguistic forms, they may have touched those parts of the psycholinguistic system that syntactically focused therapies cannot reach.

References

Bates E, Chen S, Tzeng O, Li P, Opie M (1991) The noun-verb problem in Chinese aphasia. Brain and Language 41: 203–33.
Berndt RS, Haendiges AN, Mitchum CC, Sandson J (1997a) Verb retrieval in aphasia: 1 Characterising single word impairments. Brain and Language 56: 68–106.
Berndt RS, Haendiges AN, Mitchum CC, Sandson J (1997b) Verb retrieval in aphasia: 2 Relationship to sentence processing. Brain and Language 56: 107–37.
Black M, Nickels L, Byng S (1991) Patterns of sentence processing deficit: processing simple sentences can be a complex matter. Journal of Neurolinguistics 6: 79–101.
Bloom L (1970) Language Development: Form and Function in Emerging Grammars. Cambridge, MA: MIT Press.
Bowerman M (1996) The origins of children's spatial semantic categories: cognitive versus linguistic determinants. In Gumperz JJ, Levinson SC, (Eds) Rethinking Linguistic Relativity. Cambridge: Cambridge University Press. pp145–76.
Braine MDS (1976) Children's first word combinations. Monographs of the Society of Research in Child Development 41, Serial no. 164.
Breedin SD, Saffran EM, Coslett HB (1994) Reversal of the concreteness effect in a patient with semantic dementia. Cognitive Neuropsychology 11: 617–60.
Breedin SD, Saffran EM, Schwartz MF (1998) Semantic factors in verb retrieval: an effect of complexity. Brain and Language 63: 1–31.

Brown R (1973) A First Language: The Early Stages. Cambridge: Harvard University Press.

Byng S (1988) Sentence processing deficits: theory and therapy. Cognitive Neuropsychology 5: 629–76.

Byng S, Black M (1989) Some aspects of sentence production in aphasia. Aphasiology 3: 241–63.

Byng S, Nickels L, Black M (1994) Replicating therapy for mapping deficits in agrammatism: remapping the deficit? Aphasiology 8: 315–41.

Caramazza A, Hillis A (1991) Lexical organization of nouns and verbs in the brain. Nature 349: 788–90.

Caramazza A, Miozzo M (1997) The relation between syntactic and phonological knowledge in lexical access: evidence from the tip-of-the-tongue phenomenon. Cognition 64: 309–43.

Chiat S (2000) Understanding Children with Language Problems. Cambridge: Cambridge University Press.

Choi S (1997) Language-specific input and early semantic development: evidence from children learning Korean. In Slobin DI, (Ed) The Crosslinguistic Study of Language Acquisition, Vol. 5. Mahwah, NJ: Lawrence Erlbaum Associates.

Clark EV (1993) The Lexicon in Acquisition. Cambridge: Cambridge University Press.

Cupples L, Inglis AL (1993) When task demands induce 'asyntactic' comprehension: a study of sentence interpretation in aphasia. Cognitive Neuropsychology 10: 201–34.

Devescovi A, Bates E, D'Amico S, Hernandez A, Marangolo P, Pizzamiglio L, Razzano C (1997) An on-line study of grammaticality judgements in normal and aphasic speakers of Italian. Aphasiology 11: 543–79.

Dipper LT (1999) Event Processing for Language: An Investigation of the Relationship Between Events, Sentences and Verbs, Using Data From 6 People with Non-fluent Aphasia. Unpublished PhD Dissertation. University College, London.

Evelyn M (1996) An Investigation of Verb Processing in a Child with a Specific Language Impairment. Unpublished MPhil thesis. City University, London.

Fisher C, Hall G, Rakowitz S, Gleitman L (1994) When it is better to receive than to give: syntactic and conceptual constraints on vocabulary growth. Lingua 92: 333–75.

Frawley W (1992) Linguistic Semantics. Hillsdale, NJ: Lawrence Erlbaum.

Friederici AD, Frazier, L (1992) Thematic analysis in agrammatic comprehension – syntactic structures and task demands. Brain and Language 42: 1–29.

Gentner D (1982) Why nouns are learned before verbs: linguistic relativity versus natural partitioning. In Kuczaj S, (Ed) Language Development, Vol. 2: Language, Thought, and Culture. Hillsdale, NJ: Lawrence Erlbaum Associates.

Gentner D, Medina J (1998) Similarity and the development of rules. Cognition 65: 263–97.

Gleitman LR, Gillette J (1995) The role of syntax in verb learning. In Fletcher P, MacWhinney B, (Eds) The Handbook of Child Language. Oxford: Blackwell. pp 413–27.

Gumperz JJ, Levinson SC (Eds) (1996) Rethinking Linguistic Relativity. Cambridge: Cambridge University Press.

Haendiges AN, Berndt RS, Mitchum CC (1996) Assessing the elements contributing to a 'mapping' deficit: a targeted treatment study. Brain and Language 52: 276–302.

Hillis A, Caramazza A (1995) Representation of grammatical knowledge in the brain. Journal of Cognitive Neuroscience 7: 396–407.

Jackendoff R (1983) Semantics and Cognition. Cambridge, MA: MIT Press.

Jackendoff R (1990) Semantic Structures. Cambridge, MA: MIT Press.

Jackendoff R (1997) The Architecture of the Language Faculty. Cambridge, MA: MIT Press.

Jones EV (1984) Word order processing in aphasia: effect of verb semantics. In Rose FC, (Ed) Advances in Neurology, Vol. 42: Progress in Aphasiology. New York: Raven.

Jones EV (1986) Building the foundations for sentence production in a non-fluent aphasic. British Journal of Disorders of Communication 21: 63–82.

Jörg S, Hörmann H (1978) The influence of general and specific verbal labels on the recognition of pictures. Journal of Verbal Learning and Verbal Behaviour 17: 445–55.

Langacker RW (1997) The contextual basis of cognitive semantics. In Nuyts J, Pederson E, (Eds) Language and Conceptualisation. Cambridge: Cambridge University Press.

Leonard L (1998) Children with Specific Language Impairment. Cambridge, MA: MIT Press.

Levelt WJM (1996) Perspective taking and ellipsis in spatial descriptions. In Bloom P, Peterson M, Nadel L, Garrett M, (Eds) Language and Space. Cambridge, MA: MIT Press.

Levelt WJM, Roelofs A, Meyer AS (1999) A theory of lexical access in speech production. Behavioural and Brain Sciences 22: 1–38.

Marshall J, Black M, Byng S (1999) Working with Sentences: A Handbook for Aphasia Therapists. London: Winslow Press.

Marshall J, Chiat S, Pring T (1997) An impairment of processing verbs' thematic roles: a therapy study. Aphasiology 11: 855–76.

Marshall J, Chiat S, Robson J, Pring T (1996) Calling a salad a federation: an investigation of semantic jargon, Part 2 – Verbs. Journal of Neurolinguistics 9: 251–60.

Marshall J, Pring T, Chiat S (1993) Sentence processing therapy: working at the level of the event. Aphasiology 7: 177–99.

Marshall J, Pring T, Chiat S (1998) Verb retrieval and sentence production in aphasia. Brain and Language 63: 159–83.

McCarthy R, Warrington EK (1985) Category specificity in an agrammatic patient: the relative impairment of verb retrieval and comprehension. Neuropsychologia 23: 709–27.

Meyer AS, Sleiderink AM, Levelt WJM (1998). Viewing and naming objects. Cognition 66: B25–33.

Miceli G, Silveri MC, Nocentini U, Caramazza A (1984) Patterns of dissociation in comprehension and production of nouns and verbs. Aphasiology 2: 351–58.

Mitchum CC, Berndt RS (1994) Verb retrieval and sentence construction: effects of targeted intervention. In Humphreys GW, Riddoch JM, (Eds) Cognitive Neuropsychology and Cognitive Rehabilitation. London: Erlbaum. pp 317–48.

Mitchum CC, Haendiges AN, Berndt RS (1993) Model-guided treatment to improve written sentence production: a case study. Aphasiology 7: 71–109.

Naigles LR, Eisenberg AR, Kako ET, Highter M, McGraw N (1998) Speaking of motion. Language and Cognitive Processes 13: 521–49.

Nelson K (1973) Structure and strategy in learning to talk. Monographs of the Society for Research in Child Development 38, serial no 149: 1–136.

Nickels L, Byng S, Black M (1991) Sentence processing deficits: a replication of therapy. The British Journal of Disorders of Communication 26: 175–201.

Pinker S (1989) Learnability and Cognition: The Acquisition of Argument Structure. Cambridge, MA: MIT Press.

Rapp B, Caramazza A (1997) The modality-specific organization of grammatical categories: evidence from impaired spoken and written sentence production. Brain and Language 56: 248–86.

Rice ML, Bode JV (1993) GAPS in the verb lexicons of children with specific language impairment. First Language 13: 113–31.

Schwartz M, Linebarger M, Saffran EM (1985) The status of the syntactic deficit theory of agrammatism. In Kean M-L, (Ed) Agrammatism. Orlando, FA: Academic Press.

Schwartz M, Saffran EM, Fink RB, Myers JL, Martin N (1994) Mapping therapy: A treatment programme for agrammatism. Aphasiology 8: 19–54.

Schwartz M, Saffran EM, Marin O (1980) The word order problem in agrammatism, 1 Comprehension. Brain and Language 10: 249–62.

Slobin DI (1973) Cognitive prerequisites for the acquisition of grammar. In Ferguson CA, Slobin DI, (Eds) Studies of Child Language Development. New York: Holt, Rinehart and Winston.

Slobin DI (1996) From 'thought and language' to 'thinking for speaking'. In Gumperz JJ, Levinson SC, (Eds) Rethinking Linguistic Relativity. Cambridge: Cambridge University Press. pp 70–96.

Sridhar SN (1988) Cognition and Sentence Production: A Cross-linguistic Study. New York: Springer Verlag.

Tomasello M (1995) Joint attention as social cognition. In Moore C, Dunham PJ, (Eds) Joint Attention: Its Origins and Role in Development. Hillsdale, NJ: Lawrence Erlbaum.

Tomasello M, Akhtar N, Dodson K, Rekau L (1997) Differential productivity in young children's use of nouns and verbs. Journal of Child Language 24: 373–87.

Tomlin RS (1997) Mapping conceptual representations into linguistic representations: the role of attention in grammar. In Nuyts J, Pederson E, (Eds) Language and Conceptualisation. Cambridge: Cambridge University Press.

Watkins RV, Rice ML, Moltz CC (1993) Verb use by language-impaired and normally developing children. First Language 13: 133–43.

Williams SE, Canter CJ (1987) Action-naming performance in four syndromes of aphasia. Brain and Language 32: 124–36.

Zingeser LB, Berndt RS (1990) Retrieval of nouns and verbs in agrammatism and anomia. Brain and Language 29: 14–32.

CHAPTER 4

Category-specific semantic disorders

WENDY BEST

Introduction

Warrington (1975) describes three people with 'selective impairment of semantic memory'. All had diffuse cerebral lesions. One of them, AB, was better at giving definitions to abstract than to concrete words. For example, when asked about *acorn* he replied. 'I don't know'. In contrast, *supplication* was described as 'making a serious request for help'. This remarkable dissociation pioneered a whole series of studies on category-specific semantic deficits. In AB's case the discrepancy was between concrete and abstract items. In the majority of cases described in this chapter there is a discrepancy in performance between living and non-living things.

Warrington discusses the results of her study in terms of a semantic memory impairment with a verbal memory impairment stemming from this. She also contrasts these people, with semantic memory impairments, with cases of amnesia in whom semantic memory is intact and episodic memory is impaired.

She used probe questions at different levels of specificity (e.g. Is it an animal? Is it foreign? Is it bigger than a cat?) with either a picture or a spoken word provided. Warrington argues that the results for all three cases represent evidence for hierarchical organization of semantic memory in that they show preservation of broad category information and relative vulnerability of specific information.

Research into disorders of semantic memory and, in particular, disorders that are specific to a category is very important in attempting to understand how our conceptual knowledge is structured. Several models of semantic organization have been outlined in Chapter 1 of the book and we have looked at implemented connectionist models of semantics in

Chapter 2. Here, therefore, the focus is on descriptions of single case studies with passing reference to models covered in detail elsewhere in the book. In formulating such models it is essential to use converging evidence from studies carried out with people without brain damage as well as with people with category-specific disorders following damage.

This chapter outlines a series of single cases where difficulties are experienced with a set (or sets) of items while other categories are (sometimes relatively) preserved across a variety of tasks. A comprehensive view of all reported cases is beyond the scope of this chapter. (A special issue of the journal *Neurocase*, in 1998, lists information on over 50 cases with category-specific semantic deficits.) The focus here is on selected cases that highlight specific points or stages in the development of research in the area. The aim is to provide a flavour of category-specific deficits and to illustrate some important methodological issues.

This chapter covers several descriptions, from the 1980s, of people who were impaired on processing living items relative to non-living. This is followed by two possible alternative explanations for these deficits. Both claim that the impairments are not in fact category specific but instead reflect the influence of important variables (visual complexity/ overlap and familiarity) that have not been properly controlled. Studies describing cases with the reverse dissociation, an impairment for artefacts (non-living things), are described. Next, cases held to have 'post-semantic' semantic category deficits are outlined (and largely dismissed). The chapter then focuses on more recent studies of category-specific deficits where researchers have looked in detail at deficits and strengths in 'attribute knowledge' within semantic categories. Finally the (rather limited) research into rehabilitation of category-specific deficits is summarized. The chapter ends by highlighting key methodological issues.

The chapter does not cover non-semantic category-specific deficits, for example deficits specific to proper names/word classes. In addition, there is little mention of neural localization of the deficits. It is only as better controlled studies of category-specific disorders emerge that brain imaging studies may then combine with these to produce fruitful results. (See Caramazza and Shelton, 1998, footnote 29, where strong criticisms which highlight this point are made of a recent imaging study by Damasio, Grabowski et al.,1996.) Thus the arguments here pertain to functional processing and not neural processing.

Throughout the chapter a broad distinction is made between impairment of living things (e.g. animals, fruit, vegetables) and non-living things or artefacts (e.g. tools, furniture, clothing). However, it will become clear that category-specific deficits rarely respect this strict living/non-living distinction completely (for discussion of this issue see Caramazza and Shelton, 1998).

Impairments of living things

In a series of early papers several people were described who were impaired on tasks involving animate items while performing well with inanimate things (Sartori and Job, 1988; Silveri and Gainotti, 1988; Warrington and Shallice, 1984). All of these cases had suffered from herpes simplex encephalitis. They were impaired at visual object recognition and at naming objects to verbal definition as well as to visual presentation.

Warrington and Shallice describe two people, JBR and SBY, both worse at naming and identifying living things than inanimate objects. In fact, JBR was not just poor on animate items but also failed to define musical instruments, names of fabrics or precious stones (experiment 8; SBY was not tested in this experiment). There was consistency within modality, but not across modality. The authors argue there are at least two modality-specific semantic systems. One of these would be based on functional specifications for inanimate objects – i.e. what an item is used for – and the other on sensory features for living things (and other items more easily differentiated by sensory features, such as gems).

Sensory/functional theory versus domain-specific knowledge

Warrington and Shallice's theory of the organization of semantic memory has been interpreted in different ways (see Chapter 1). The most influential interpretation has been that animate items are differentially impaired when there is a lesion involving visual semantic representations because our understanding of such items relies heavily on their visual characteristics (e.g. leopards have spots, oranges are orange). In contrast, a lesion involving functional semantic representations would differentially impair performance on inanimate objects because these tend to rely on function for their meaning (e.g. pens are for writing).

On this interpretation of the theory, category-specific impairments are not really category specific at all but reduce to the fact that animate and inanimate items rely differentially on visual and functional features for their meaning. As these areas of semantics are damaged, so dissociations between categories 'fall out' depending on the reliance of the items on different types of information. Caramazza and Shelton (1998) term this reductionist account of category-specific deficits the 'sensory functional theory' (also referred to as the 'differential weighting hypothesis'; Lambon Ralph, Howard, Nightingale et al., 1998). Caramazza and Shelton contrast this with their preferred account in which knowledge is 'domain specific', i.e. is categorically organized into broad domains along lines which reflect evolutionary salience (see Chapter 1 for details).

A modality- and category-specific deficit?

A man (TOB) described by McCarthy and Warrington (1988) was also disproportionately impaired on living things. His speech was fluent with evidence of word finding difficulties. He suffered progressive deterioration due to an abnormality in the left temporal lobe. TOB was impaired at naming and matching spoken words to pictures for living things. He could, however, obtain meaning from pictures of living things. For example, he could give semantic information from pictures, including verbal information (e.g. that a rhinoceros lives in Africa). The authors argue that TOB's deficit provides evidence for dissociable modality-specific meaning systems, and that his verbal knowledge is impaired within one semantic category. This seems odd in the light of the fact that he could provide verbal information about pictures of animate items. This paper provides an example of the confusion over the term 'modality' in this area of research. As Coltheart, Inglis, Cupples et al., (1998) point out, 'modality' may refer to the nature of sensory input (mode of presentation) or to the type of semantic knowledge (e.g. visual versus functional knowledge).

Naming to definition: varying the type of information

Silveri and Gainotti (1988) describe LA who showed a pattern of impairment similar to the people described by Warrington and Shallice (1984). There were category-specific problems with animals, fruit and flowers and with foods, but good performance with body parts. She was poor at naming to 'visual' definitions – 1/11 (e.g. an insect with broad coloured ornate wings) but good with 'verbal' definitions – 8/14 (e.g. a farm animal that bellows and supplies us with milk). However, Stewart, Parkin and Hunkin (1992) point out that the mean word frequency for the two sets differed (visual, 5.3; verbal, 21.1), suggesting the effect maybe due to frequency rather than semantic category. (See below for further discussion of this issue and further work with LA.) She was consistent within and across modalities (although this may also reflect an underlying frequency effect) and the authors use this to argue for the existence of a single semantic system.

Alternative explanations for semantic category deficits

Having provided a description of some reports of category-specific deficits from the 1980s, we now consider objections to the claim that the impairments are really specific to semantic category. It may be that these cases are sensitive to a particular variable that characterizes stimuli from a category but that is not particular to that category. Two possible underlying variables are discussed: visual complexity/overlap and familiarity.

Visual explanation of category effects

This is different from the sensory functional hypothesis which claims that the effects arise because categories rely differentially on types of knowledge within the semantic system. In contrast, the visual explanation of category-specific effects expounded here holds that the impairment is not within central semantics but is within the structural description system (Chapter 1). The problem is specific to modality of input (cf. optic aphasia discussed in Chapter 1). As categories of natural items tend to have higher levels of perceptual overlap between exemplars than categories of artefactual objects (Humphreys, Riddoch, and Quinlan, 1988), this deficit would differentially impair performance on living categories. The key task here is the object decision test (analogous to lexical decision) which has been used as the standard test of access to structural descriptions (Riddoch and Humphreys, 1993). If someone is able to do this task it suggests that pre-semantic visual processing is intact. If someone is unable to do this task an apparently 'semantic' deficit may arise, as the impairment in structural descriptions is likely to impair performance with living items more than non-living.

This problem is exemplified by a case described by Sartori and Job (1988). Michelangelo was better at naming objects than animals, fruit or vegetables. On an object decision task he accepted real animals and objects but also accepted many non-objects and animals. He also gave impaired descriptions from the names of animate objects because, the authors suggest, 'structural descriptions also mediate the verbal production of visual features' (p 130). Michelangelo could, however, judge correctly categorical relations, ferocity, animal sounds and environments which are argued to tap semantic information without involvement of structural descriptions.

The authors conclude that his impairment is at the level of structural descriptions (specific to the categories for which he has problems) and that it is from here that a visual description arises (Sartori and Job, 1988: 128). Likewise, Coltheart et al. (1998) claim that structural descriptions are used for (a) recognizing visually presented objects; (b) when answering questions about the visual attributes of objects; and also possibly (c) when drawing. It is impossible, in this case, to maintain the distinction between structural descriptions (used purely for recognition) and visual semantic knowledge. If 'structural descriptions' form part of semantic knowledge then the visual explanation for category-specific effects translates into the following: within semantics the representations for living things tend to have higher levels of overlap with each other, thus general damage to visual semantic representations will selectively impair performance on living things. While this account of impairments does not rely on animate items depending more heavily on visual than functional features for their meaning (Farah and McClelland, 1991), it parallels the sensory functional theory in that category-specific deficits are not genuinely category specific but rather 'fall out' of underlying attributes (the visual similarity/dissimilarity) of category members. Note, however, that in the case of Michelangelo, Sartori and Job are claiming a category-specific problem within structural descriptions. Further detailed studies of people with category-specific deficits but without problems with object decision are necessary to disentangle this issue. Additionally, in making claims about category-specific effects in object decision, investigators need to control for the levels of perceptual overlap of items combined to form the non-objects across living and non-living categories. Obviously, as there tends to be more visual overlap with other category members for living than non-living things, it will be hard to control the real items on this variable. There are no studies where such care has been taken and many that report a deficit on this task. For example, the commonly used BORB object decision task (Riddoch and Humphreys, 1993) contains many more animate than inanimate items.

Familiarity explanation of category effects

Funnell and Sheridan (1992) suggest item familiarity may underlie apparent category-specific effects. They describe the performance of a young woman, SL, who had suffered a head injury. Initial testing showed an impairment on living things with respect to non-living things. However, in a second picture-naming experiment they pitted category type against familiarity. The results show that the apparent category effects were in fact an artefact of differences in the familiarity of the original items in the sets of living and non-living things.

In addition, Funnell and Sheridan (1992) show that, in the widely used Snodgrass and Vanderwart (1980) pictures, living things are generally of lower familiarity than non-living. On re-analysing the data from JBR (Warrington and Shallice, 1984; experiment 7), Funnell and Sheridan found that his performance correlated with familiarity and argue that this may explain away anomalies in the categories that are impaired. For example, JBR performed well with body parts, which is out of keeping with his poor performance on other animate items; body parts are high in familiarity. In contrast he was poor with musical instruments while performing well with other inanimate categories; musical instruments are low in familiarity. Funnell and Sheridan argue that, once familiarity is taken into account, there is no convincing evidence for the organization of semantic memory into living and non-living things.

Funnell and De Mornay Davies (1996) reassessed JBR (one of the people originally described by Warrington and Shallice, 1984). They found that he did have a genuine impairment on living things but that this was restricted to low familiarity items. In addition, control participants showed a tendency to be worse with living things. The authors suggest that the nature of JBR's deficit is not pathological but concede that the degree of his deficit for living things is abnormal.

In a similar vein to Funnell and Sheridan, Stewart, Parkin and Hunkin (1992) show that controlling for familiarity removed an apparent category-specific naming impairment in case HO (who was impaired on naming animals and musical instruments). They suggest that it is important to control for frequency, familiarity and visual complexity when investigating category-specific effects.

Category-specific effects over and above the influence of familiarity

There are, however, several studies where category-specific disorders for living things remain even when familiarity is taken into account (e.g. Caramazza and Shelton, 1998; Forde, Francis, Riddoch et al., 1997; Laiacona, Barbarotto and Capitani, 1993; Lambon Ralph, Howard, Nightingale et al., 1998; Moss, Tyler and Jennings, 1997; Gainotti and Silveri, 1996).

For example, Gainotti and Silveri (1996) carried out further studies with LA. They demonstrated that her naming was worse for living items even when familiarity was controlled. However, her naming was also influenced by familiarity. Interestingly, body parts were also spared whereas naming of 'food' and 'musical instruments' were severely impaired. On a new naming to definition task (naming the same stimuli once from perceptual and once from functional information), LA was worst at naming living things from perceptual information. However, she also showed a general impairment on naming living things relative to non-living. This effect was not shown by the controls who did, however, tend to be worse at generating names in response to perceptual than to functional definitions.

Thus, the strong claim of Funnell and Sheridan (1992) that variables such as familiarity may underlie all category-specific effects has not been upheld by subsequent studies. However, the work was crucial in highlighting the need for research to control such variables as, in a number of cases, these are likely to underlie the apparent category-specific impairment.

Impairments of non-living things

By far the majority of cases of category-specific deficit that have been reported have involved an impairment of living things relative to non-living. However, the reverse dissociation has also been found occasionally. (For example, in the *Neurocase* special issue of 1998 there were listed over 50 cases of impairment for living things and only 7 cases with a specific impairment for non-living things.) This finding of an impairment for non-living things is very important for a number of reasons:

a) It provides a double dissociation (Shallice, 1988) with the more common finding of a deficit on living things. Thus it is not the case that living things are simply 'more difficult' in some unspecified way. This allows for claims about functional organization of the semantic system.

b) It provides further evidence against the claim that category-specific deficits are all attributable to some underlying variables (such as familiarity or visual overlap of items within a category). However, it does not exclude the possibility that both types of category-specific deficit are artefactual albeit for different reasons; the reverse impairment may simply reflect different underlying variables (a possibility not considered by many authors, e.g. Saffran and Schwartz, 1994).

c) It allows for the same stimuli and tasks to be used with people with opposing patterns of deficit (Hillis and Caramazza, 1991; Lambon Ralph et al., 1998). Such studies are immune to some of the criticisms directed at studies of category-specific impairments and therefore should take us further in understanding what such deficits reveal about the organization of meaning.

Non-living items tend to be of higher familiarity than living. Logically, this suggests that when familiarity is controlled, some cases may turn out to be better with animate than inanimate items (the difference usually being obscured by familiarity differences built into the testing materials). Howard, Best, Bruce and Gatehouse (1995) worked with several people with aphasia. When familiarity, length, frequency, age of acquisition, imageability and concreteness were controlled, one member of the group was significantly better at naming animate than inanimate items. However, in his case, further investigations showed this apparent category effect was due to better performance with items known to multiple senses.

In general, the early cases of poor performance with living items relative to non-living were found in post-encephalitic cases and not in people with aphasia due to stroke or head injury. The reverse pattern, better performance with living things, has been found mainly in people who are severely aphasic. For example, Warrington and McCarthy (1987) describe the performance of YOT, who had suffered an extensive left hemisphere lesion and was globally aphasic. He performed better with animals and foods than objects, on a fast word to picture matching task. With a delay between the picture and spoken input, he was equally good with all the items. Further categories were also examined: e.g. performance was better with large outdoor objects (e.g. vehicles and buildings) than with small manipulable objects. The authors suggest that the dissociation in performance should not be considered with respect to animacy, but in terms of the sensory/functional distinction; large items are usually observed visually while smaller items are more likely to be manipulated.

A striking case of the reverse dissociation

Sacchett and Humphreys (1992) describe CW who showed a deficit for naming and comprehension of artefactual objects and body parts with preservation of natural items (animals, foods). This discrepancy occurred even though the non-living things and body parts used in one naming experiment were rated as more familiar and less visually complex than the 'natural objects'. The discrepancy between performance on living and non-living things was striking. For example, CW named 95% of living things and only 35% of non-living things.

Sparing of or damage to a semantic property?

Finally, cases described by Hillis and Caramazza (1991) are outlined. One, JJ, who had suffered a left temporal lobe infarct, showed very good spoken and written naming, comprehension and definition of animals (and transport) relative to other categories. The errors on naming tasks were mainly semantic co-ordinates. The authors argue that JJ shows performance consistent with central semantic damage. They suggest that he may have relative sparing of a semantic feature common to animal and transport categories (such as mobility). The reverse pattern was shown by PS, who had suffered a head injury. He was held to have a selective deficit of the 'mobility' feature. This interpretation relates well to Allport's (1985) model of semantic memory (see Chapter 1 and Coltheart et al., 1998). In Allport's distributed model a single item will be represented by a set of auto-associated activity patterns which span modalities (sensory and motor) in which it has meaning. Although the suggestion by Hillis and Caramazza that the 'feature' mobility is impaired seems, at first, highly specific it may be possible to marry this claim with this type of model. Perhaps mobility is represented in a sub-area of Allport's action-orientated elements. In this case, damage to this area would impair this aspect of meaning for all mobile items. However, if this is the only damage that has occurred, then PP should be good at judging other aspects of meaning, e.g. the shape of animals and vehicles or the noises that they make, and PP was not tested on such features.

In summary, several cases have now been reported where performance on living things is better than on non-living; the reverse dissociation from the early cases showing category-specific deficits for living things. The cases taken together provide a double dissociation, showing that it is not simply that one category is harder to process than the other. In every case, however, it is important to ensure that the effect genuinely reflects semantic category and not the influence of another variable (such as familiarity for those better with living things or age of acquisition for those better with non-living things). These cases demonstrate the need for models of conceptual knowledge that can be damaged so as to impair meaning of either living or non-living items.

Post-semantic semantic category deficits?

We shall now consider two cases held to have category-specific deficits occurring at a post-semantic level.

Hart et al., (1985) describe a case (MD) who was not clinically aphasic on the Boston Diagnostic Aphasia Examination. MD was unable to name fruit or vegetables but showed good comprehension of these items. Taking frequency (but not familiarity) into account did not explain the category-specific effect on naming. He was poor with fruit and vegetables on a variety of tasks: naming to definition, touch, verbal fluency, and also picture categorization. In contrast, he was unimpaired on word to picture matching and judgements regarding properties of fruit and vegetables. They argue his case shows that the output lexicon is addressed by semantically categorized information that can be disrupted highly selectively. This does not, however, explain the poor performance on picture categorization. It would be useful to have more information on MD's comprehension e.g. response times for word to picture matching of fruit and vegetables versus other categories. This is particularly relevant as the authors note that MD was hesitant for fruit and vegetables on the comprehension task. Perhaps, although more evident in tasks requiring output, his central semantic representations for fruit and vegetables are impaired and thorough testing of comprehension would reveal a difference between categories.

Similarly, Farah and Wallace (1992) describe a case (TU) who had problems naming fruit and vegetables. This was the case regardless of whether naming was required in response to object, picture or definition. Spoken naming was also influenced by familiarity and by frequency. The authors argue that TU has intact comprehension for these items, for example, once given a name, he could give a good description of the item. Apart from this, the tests for comprehension were not very stringent. For example, TU was given a choice of three names to go with an object. He was correct on 22/24 items. He might, however, have been using a process of elimination. Judgement of whether a single name was correct for the object (Howard and Orchard-Lisle, 1984) would have been a more stringent assessment. TU's errors on attempting to name fruit and vegetables were mostly semantic.

The authors argue that TU's deficit is in the process by which phonology is accessed from semantics for output. However, Farah and Wallace note that the consistency in TU's performance suggests impaired representations (rather than access). They propose a layer of hidden units may correspond to semantically similar words and that at least some of the representations needed for naming are implemented in a relatively local manner (see Chapter 5). In order to be convincing, Hart et al. and Farah and Wallace need to use comprehension tasks that are not performed at ceiling (e.g. using reaction times) and then show that no category-specific effect exists.

Varying the modality of input

As we have seen, studies in this area tend to compare performance across verbal and pictorial input when attempting to draw conclusions about the nature of a person's deficit and underlying semantic organization. Other studies have taken this further and looked at performance in response to environmental sounds (e.g. Caramazza and Shelton, 1998; Coltheart et al., 1998) and to touch and taste (e.g. Forde et al., 1997). Such investigations are important in considering claims about modality (of knowledge) specific semantic subsystems. As an example, consider the naming data and the authors' interpretation of the deficit of SBR (Forde at al., 1997, described again in the section on rehabilitation later in the chapter). SBR had suffered a haemorrhage as a result of an underlying arteriovenous malformation. He was worse at naming pictures of living than non-living things. This extended to naming real objects from vision. He was also asked to name from touch. Here performance on non-living objects was at ceiling. In contrast he named only 3/9 fruit and vegetables. This was significantly worse than control performance as was his naming of fruit and vegetables from taste. Naming to definition was significantly worse than controls for auditory definitions based on visual-perceptual properties but was good for functional-encyclopaedic definitions; there was no semantic category effect on this task. Forde at al. (1997) claim that SBR has a general deficit in a (non-categorical) structural description system. This deficit has a particular effect on structurally similar categories such as fruit and vegetables. Why, in this case, would SBR exhibit category-specific deficits across modalities of input other than vision? The researchers must hold, although this is not explicit in the paper, the idea that naming from other modalities of input necessitates reliance on visual structural descriptions.

Investigation of naming from a variety of modalities of input may help clarify the nature of category-specific deficits and the claims that are being made in relation to models of conceptual organization.

Investigations of attribute knowledge

In the studies described so far, investigators have used a variety of tasks such as naming of pictures and naming to definition to tap semantic knowledge. As studies of category-specific deficits evolve, researchers are looking in more detail at the specific feature knowledge available within the living and non-living categories. If, for example, someone is unable to name pictures of a table or a pig, what knowledge do they retain about these items? This can be investigated using forced choice questions, such as 'Do they have legs?' or 'What category are they from?' In this section the term 'attribute' is used broadly to incorporate knowledge about any aspect or feature of meaning. 'Attributes' are subdivided into three types of property: superordinate category knowledge (e.g. a dog is an animal, a chair is a piece of furniture); perceptual knowledge (e.g. a dog has legs, a chair has legs), and associative/functional knowledge (e.g. dogs can bark, chairs are for sitting on).

One way of considering the data is in the light of two theories of semantic organization which make contrasting predictions. The first, described above, is the sensory functional theory, which holds that the apparent category-specific deficits reduce to the degree to which categories rely on sensory versus functional properties (see also Chapter 1). In this case if there is damage to sensory properties, while living categories may be more impaired, there will also be some effect on non-living things. In particular there will be evidence of an impairment of sensory knowledge of non-living things (Farah and McClelland, 1991; Warrington and McCarthy, 1987). A contrasting hypothesis holds that the category-specific effects are genuine and reflect specific domains of semantic knowledge (Caramazza and Shelton, 1998: see Chapter 1, this book). In this case an impairment in processing living things may be restricted to this domain and there need be no necessary accompanying impairment in sensory knowledge of non-living things.

Laiacona et al. (1993) carried out the first well controlled studies in this area. They worked with two people (FM and RG) who had suffered head injuries. Both demonstrated a selective impairment for naming and comprehension of living things, which remained after a number of variables including frequency, familiarity and visual complexity were partialed out. Interestingly, controls were also worse at naming living (67% correct) than non-living (87% correct) things. The difference for FM and RG remained significant when control performance was taken into account. In addition, in responding to semantic feature questions, neither FM nor RG exhibited a difference between perceptual and associative knowledge. For example, FM performed within normal limits on both visual and functional property questions for non-living things. In contrast, in relation to living things, he was 72% correct for both visual and associative properties. Thus, 'preferential impairment of perceptual information is not necessary for the emergence of a selective impairment for living things' (Laiacona et al., 1993: 378). This appears to provide fairly strong evidence against the sensory functional theory, which holds that the category effect for living things arises from deficits in underlying sensory representations. If this was true, FM and RG should show a differential impairment for sensory representation of living things and also a relative impairment in sensory knowledge (over associative knowledge) for non-living things. This was not found.

There is, however, a potential problem with the methodology of the paper: the 6 attribute questions for each item were presented on the same occasion and in the same order (superordinate – 2; perceptual – 2; and associative – 2). If priming of semantic knowledge is occurring (Moss et al., 1997), this may influence the outcome; for example, intact superordinate knowledge may have primed knowledge of other attributes. In the case of FM and RG the problem is somewhat alleviated by the fact the perceptual questions (presumed impaired on the sensory functional account of deficits for living things) were presented prior to the attribute questions, and that the cross-category difference was so strong. A difference between types of attribute knowledge (e.g. perceptual>associative) would be hard to interpret using this order of questions.

This finding has been replicated more recently in two people after they had had herpes simplex encephalitis (Laiacona, Capitani and Barbarotto, 1997). Therefore, even in people with the same neurological aetiology as the early cases of category-specific semantic disorders, a discrepancy between visual and functional knowledge does not necessarily occur. Importantly, in both cases, object decision was performed well, suggesting the impairment in these people was in central semantic representations rather than structural descriptions.

Priming of attribute knowledge

Investigations of attribute knowledge were also carried out with SE (Moss et al., 1997). The paper is of interest because it describes a priming study in someone with a category-specific deficit. SE had a provisional diagnosis of herpes simplex encephalitis. He was originally described by Laws, Evans, Hodges et al. (1995) who claimed to have found that he had a category-specific deficit for living things with a selective problem with non-visual associative properties of living things.

First, Moss at al. (1997) demonstrated that SE had a mild category-specific deficit for living things. His definitions for single words were rated more highly for non-living than living things. This effect remained when a subset of items matched for familiarity was analysed. His picture naming, on sets matched for familiarity and visual complexity, was also worse for living than non-living things. In an experiment involving semantic priming of lexical decision, the controls showed priming for visual and non-visual primes and no difference between the living and non-living categories. Moss et al. (1997) used this online task with SE with the aim of revealing impairments that might be compensated for by additional processing in offline tasks. SE showed priming overall, but when the target was a visual property of the prime, he showed priming for the non-living (e.g. harp–strings) but not for the living category (e.g. fox–red). SE was also tested using an offline property verification task. As well as manipulating category and type of property (visual/non-visual), the distinctiveness of properties was manipulated. (E.g. 'tigers have legs' is a general property as many animals have legs; in contrast, 'tigers have stripes' is a distinctive property as only a few animals have stripes). SE performed well overall. However, he did show significantly worse performance on living things and this was particularly marked for the distinctive properties (see also data for EW: Caramazza and Shelton, 1998). No control participant showed this pattern.

SE's definitions were analysed again, in more detail, and compared with those from controls. Performance was within the normal range for non-living things and for non-visual properties of living things. However, as in the other two tasks, he showed a specific deficit with the visual properties of living things.

The discrepancy between this finding and that of Laws et al. (1995), who claim to have shown SE has a deficit for associative properties of living things, is discussed in some detail in the paper. In brief, Moss et al. claim that a wide range of materials and detailed comparisons with controls are necessary to form an accurate picture of the problem.

Thus, across on- and offline tasks, SE appears to have a semantic deficit restricted to knowledge of the visual properties of living things with no impairment in the visual properties of non-living things. This finding appears at odds with the domain-specific account of semantic organization (Caramazza and Shelton, 1998) where living and non-living things are represented separately – unless subdivisions into visual and non-visual information are made within the semantic category. Additionally, the results do not fit with a simple version of the sensory functional theory, which would predict an accompanying deficit for visual attributes of non-living items. However, Moss et al. (1997) interpret the data from SE with respect to another theory, the 'intercorrelation hypothesis'. (See Chapter 5; also De Renzi and Luchelli, 1994; Gonnerman, Andersen, Devlin et al., 1997. Caramazza (1998) provides arguments against this hypothesis). They argue that the difference between living and non-living categories is the degree to which there are strong intercorrelations between form and function (or visual and non-visual properties). In the case of living things there is not generally a strong relationship. However, in the case of non-living things the shape and parts of an item can be closely tied to the function (think of hammers, trousers or bicycles). The claim is that damage to visual properties would have minimal effect on non-living things as resulting gaps in representations can be filled in by links with closely related functional properties. The argument is that SE has a general deficit for visual properties but in the case of non-living things this is compensated for by activation from the intact functional properties. In the case of living things there are only a few activation links between visual and non-visual property nodes, so the latter are unable to compensate for impairments in the former.

Thus, SE is important for a number of reasons:

a) The contrasting findings of Moss et al. (1997) and Laws et al. (1995) highlight the need for care and thoroughness in the investigation of category-specific disorders.
b) Moss et al. start with the claim that SE has a category-specific impairment for living things and then, after further investigations, claim that the deficit is for visual attributes of living things; finally, interpreting the results in relation to the intercorrelation hypothesis leads to the conclusion that he has a general (across-category) deficit for visual properties. No additional testing is carried out to investigate this claim. The need for a priori hypotheses and testing of predictions arising from these could not be clearer.
c) The results from online (priming) and offline tasks (e.g. providing definitions/judgement tasks) concur, at least for SE. This gives support to findings from offline studies being taken to reflect impaired processing without strategic compensation. However, such parallel performance may not always be found. In this case, cross-task comparisons may be especially fruitful in helping to establish the nature of the deficit and strategies that may be occurring, in some people, in offline tasks.

Further investigations of attribute knowledge

Finally, in this section, we consider three more cases where attribute knowledge has been investigated. Two cases were described by Lambon Ralph et al. (1998). They are important because they provide two (theoretically important) double dissociations. DB showed a category-specific deficit for living things whereas IW's was for non-living. In addition, they showed different patterns on tests involving attribute knowledge. DB was impaired with living things relative to non-living, regardless of whether the information required was perceptual or associative (paralleling the findings of Laiacona et al., 1993, 1997). IW was more impaired with perceptual information, and less with associative knowledge regardless of semantic category.

DB had dementia of Alzheimer's type. She showed a category-specific deficit for living things on picture naming even when the influence of a number of variables was taken into account (her naming was also influenced by object familiarity and by age of acquisition). DB, like many other people with a deficit for living things, was also impaired on object decision, although in her case the impairment was relatively mild. She achieved a score of 100/126 on a task from the BORB (Riddoch and Humphreys, 1993) where controls scored between 106 and 126. On a definition to word matching task (modified from Gainotti and Silveri, 1996) where perceptual or associative definitions were matched to one of a choice of 5 items (target and 4 semantic foils), DB was 100% on all items involving non-living things. She was 69% correct with animals in response to both perceptual and associative definitions. This pattern was mirrored on a task with semantic feature questions about 64 items. She was significantly better with non-living things than animals and there was no effect of attribute type. The 64 items in this task were 32 animals and 32 non-living things. These were matched for a number of variables (including object familiarity but excluding age of acquisition which may be important for DB). However, the paper does not present control data for this key task. It may be that controls would also find judgements about animals harder than those about attributes. This might be reflected in reaction time differences even if 100% accuracy were achieved (see discussion of methodological issues below).

Lambon Ralph et al. (1998) also worked with IW, who had semantic dementia. She tended to have slightly better performance on naming and comprehension tasks with non-living things than with living things, once important variables were well controlled. However, on the same definition to word matching task given to DB, she did not exhibit a significant difference between animals and non-living things: instead her performance was influenced by definition type. She was significantly worse with perceptual than associative definitions. Unfortunately she was not tested on the 64-item feature questions. On a feature question task, with unmatched stimuli, IW was significantly better at associative than perceptual questions but there was no effect of semantic category. Thus, her performance provides strong evidence against the sensory functional theory (differential weighting hypothesis). IW has impaired performance with perceptual attributes (relative to associative attributes) in the context of slightly (but significantly) better performance on living things in a naming task. This provides the strongest evidence yet against claims that an impairment in visual knowledge underlies category-specific impairments for living things.

Despite her relatively poor performance in matching words to visual definitions, IW performed normally on tests of object decision. (121/126 on BORB – controls, 106–126; 48/50 on a harder task – controls, 43–50). This result suggests that it is not essential to use central semantic knowledge to perform object decision; it must be possible to use other representations (which are unimpaired in IW) to perform this task.

Interestingly, DB and IW, although both impaired on drawing to dictation, showed very different patterns of performance. DB's pictures of animals and objects (while not rated differentially in relation to how good a representation of the target a picture was) were qualitatively different. The pictures of animals tended to show a 'prototype effect' regressing to the mean, e.g. with an outline of a familiar item such as cat, dog or horse. In contrast, IW's pictures missed out features, as compared with control drawings of the same items. It is not clear what is the best method for scoring drawings as there is considerable variation in the drawing abilities of the normal population. A useful comparison is between copying (to establish the effects of poor draughtsmanship), delayed copying (where no verbal input is necessary) and drawing to dictation, all in relation to the drawings of control participants (Lambon Ralph et al., 1998).

An impairment in visual attributes?

Finally, in this section, we consider the performance of AC (Coltheart et al., 1998). Like IW, AC appears to have a deficit for visual attributes without a category-specific deficit for living things. However, the two cases differ in a number of important ways.

AC had a history of cardio- and cerebrovascular disease and eventually suffered a left hemisphere stroke. After his stroke he was aphasic and had great difficulty in naming pictures. On object decision AC was impaired (45/60 and 48/60 on a pre-BORB version) with superior performance on inanimate objects. This was the only example of semantic category specificity in his performance. His knowledge of living and non-living things was tested using forced choice yes/no questions in association with a spoken object name – for example, 'Table – does it have legs?'. AC was at chance on judging a number of visual attributes (e.g. 'Does it have...legs, wheels, a tail; is it round?') regardless of whether the object was living or non-living. In contrast, he performed well on forced choice questions tapping non-perceptual attribute knowledge (e.g. 'Is it Australian? Do people usually eat it? Does it live in water?'). Thus, the authors claim that AC had little problem in dealing with non-perceptual attributes but was severely impaired with visual attributes.

Coltheart et al. (1998) went on to investigate knowledge about other sensory modalities. Using the same yes/no paradigm, AC was good at deciding which of a set of objects had characteristic smells (e.g. coffee, petrol) and at deciding which made noises (e.g. bell, flute). Thus the deficit appeared to be specific to visual attributes. When AC was given environmental sounds and asked to judge visual attributes (e.g. a train sound – 'Does it have legs?', etc.) he was again at chance.

The authors claim to have shown that AC has an impairment in retrieving visual attributes which is not modality (of input) specific. One straightforward interpretation of these findings is that AC has lost, or is unable to access, information about stored visual representations. The problem is that this interpretation depends upon his having understood the probe features (e.g. legs, wheels, etc.). In fact there are additional data suggesting that even when the picture of an item is present and shows the feature, he is impaired (e.g. animals with visible tails – 88% correct over 4 occasions; objects with visible wheels – 74% correct). This could be taken to suggest that, even with a picture present, AC does not fully understand what is being asked of him. This seems a possibility in the light of the fact that previous studies have shown that aphasic people's comprehension can be influenced by word frequency, and the key words in the sensory questions have a lower mean frequency than the key words testing associative attributes. The mean log lemma frequencies from the Celex database are: visual 1.47 (s.d. 0.68); associative 2.12 (s.d. 0.41) – excluding 'Australian' as this is likely to have a higher frequency within Australia than that suggested by the (non-Australian) database. This difference borders on significance (unrelated t-test, $t(8)=1.84$, $p>0.05$, 1-tailed).

Leaving aside such concerns, there are at least two cases where apparent difficulty with visual attributes is not accompanied by a category-specific deficit for living things (IW and AC). They provide further evidence against the sensory functional theory of category-specific deficits. So far, the reverse pattern, an isolated, disproportionate, impairment for functional over visual attributes has not been reported. It would be interesting to know whether such a problem could also dissociate from category deficits.

However, the two cases differ in a number of ways. AC had a more severe naming impairment than IW and was also impaired on object decision, a task on which IW's performance was normal. The interpretation of AC's pattern of performance is that it reflects a problem within the visual object recognition/structural description system. Coltheart et al. (1998) propose a model of semantic memory with subsystems of perceptual attribute knowledge, one for each of the different perceptual modalities, plus a system where non-perceptual knowledge is represented (Chapter 1). It is not clear how the performance of IW who had intact object decision but impaired drawing would be interpreted in relation to this model. One would have to claim that visual knowledge is intact and can be accessed to make object decisions but inaccessible for drawing and answering questions about visual attributes. Perhaps a deficit between visual knowledge and the non-perceptual semantic system on this model would allow for her pattern of performance. Lambon Ralph et al. (1998) are not entirely clear on what they consider to be the nature of IW's impairment.

Overview of studies investigating attribute knowledge

This section has described investigations of attribute knowledge in people with category-specific deficits. It will be clear from the interpretation of these different cases that they are refining theories of how conceptual knowledge is represented. In particular there is converging neuropsychological evidence which combines with the information from normal participants (Caramazza and Shelton, 1998) to refute a simple version of the sensory functional hypothesis. For example, this theory makes the strong prediction that people with category-specific deficits for living things will have an underlying deficit in visual knowledge. Cases have been shown to have a category-specific deficit for living things in the context of equally impaired performance across tasks tapping visual and associative attribute knowledge for living things and unimpaired performance on tasks tapping visual and associative knowledge of non-living things (e.g. DB: Lambon Ralph et al., 1998; Laiacona et al., 1993, 1997). In addition, there are some very specific dissociations which challenge other theories. For example, IW's intact object decision, impaired knowledge of visual attributes and drawing lacking visual features, does not sit easily with the claim by Coltheart et al. that all three tasks are performed on the basis of the visual knowledge subsystem. Also, the data showing that SE (Moss et al., 1997) has a semantic deficit restricted to the visual properties of living things challenge accounts of semantics that are organized according to semantic category (such as the domain-specific knowledge theory of Caramazza and Shelton, 1998), unless representations within these categories are also organized by type of knowledge (sensory/functional). Finally, in people with category-specific deficits for living things, naming to definition can be better when functional, rather than visual, information is provided (LA: Gainotti and Silveri, 1996; SBR: Forde et al., 1997). According to the domain-specific theory, conceptual knowledge is organized by semantic category; however, if LA and SBR have impaired representations of living things, why should their performance be influenced by the type of information used to access these concepts? It is not clear how Caramazza and Shelton (1998) can explain this pattern of performance without recourse to additional assumptions.

In summary, there are two main patterns of performance shown so far in studies using direct verbal questions designed to tap into semantic attribute knowledge. Firstly, there are cases with a category-specific deficit for living things, who show impaired knowledge of attributes for living things regardless of attribute type (EW: Caramazza and Shelton, 1998; DK: Lambon Ralph et al., 1998; Laiacona et al., 1993; 1997). These people are not impaired on attribute judgements for non-living things. Secondly, there are cases with an impairment of knowledge of sensory attributes regardless of whether the items are alive (AC: Coltheart et al., 1998; IW: Lambon Ralph et al. 1998). IW also demonstrated a category-specific deficit for non-living things once stimuli were well controlled. As more investigations using this technique emerge the patterns found should help to further elaborate models of conceptual organization. At present, however, no single model can account for all the available neuropsychological data in a straightforward manner.

Category-specific deficits – change over time

There is currently very little written on rehabilitation of people with category-specific disorders. The few studies that do exist are mixed in their conclusions. Swales and Johnson (1992) worked with JH, who had a category-specific deficit for living things after herpes simplex encephalitis. He was also amnesic for all but recent events. In the first treatment study JH was presented with a picture or word and asked to learn something about it. He was able to relearn some semantic information. The training worked best for familiar items. This suggests that information may not have been completely lost from semantic memory prior to therapy. In a second study, treatment involved identifying, writing down and learning the distinguishing features of a set of living items. After treatment JH was asked to name and provide semantic information associated with the target items. He had improved, in particular on fruit and vegetables, and this effect remained six weeks later. It would have been interesting to see whether performance generalized to untreated items sharing semantic attributes with those that were treated. The authors suggest that the retained improvement with fruit and vegetables may have been due to JH's real life exposure to these items: for instance, he was involved in cooking at home.

A rehabilitation study carried out by Sartori, Miozzo and Job (1994) came to a more depressing conclusion. They worked with Michelangelo (described above) and with Giulietta. Both had category-specific impairments for living things, and showed a deficit on tasks requiring the retrieval of perceptual knowledge such as drawing. This was accompanied by retrograde and anterograde amnesia. Treatment aimed to improve perceptual knowledge of living things. It lasted eight months and included a variety of tasks such as categorization, defining (including describing visual attributes using imagery) and drawing from memory (with a subsequent check against a picture of the object to detect errors). When retested, both individuals continued to show a marked category-specific naming impairment. Unfortunately, however, they were not tested on the same tasks pre- and post-therapy (except for naming, where a direct comparison is not given), making the authors' claims hard to evaluate. Sartori et al. argue that the treatment may have failed because of the anterograde amnesia and come to the strong conclusion that 'treatment of specific memory loss should be considered impossible if accompanied by a severe memory loss' (Sartori et al., 1994: 122).

Finally, Sheridan and Humphreys (1993) worked with a woman who was impaired with fruit and vegetables having suffered herpes simplex encephalitis. The very practical 'gastrotherapy' (using real foods) that was carried out improved her knowledge about these items while knowledge about other impaired categories remained relatively stable (Sheridan, personal communication).

Longitudinal studies without therapy

Forde at al. (1997) worked with SBR, who had a category-specific deficit for living things and was also amnesic. They dispute the conclusion of Sartori et al. (1994). While SBR's deficit was not treated, he was assessed on tasks related to his category-specific deficit for two hours per week for several months. When re-tested 12 months post-lesion, SBR was able to name most living things when given time. During this time there was very little change in his amnesia. Thus SBR's change in performance over time suggests that perceptual knowledge may improve independently of change in episodic (event) memory. Forde at al. suggest that the conclusion drawn by Sartori et al. may have been premature.

One crucial difference between the studies may be the time post-onset at which performance was first measured to compare with later performance. Unfortunately in none of these three cases (Michelangelo, Giulietta, and SBR) is the time of initial testing relative to onset clear. However, for SBR, follow-up was 12 months post-onset, suggesting the change that had occurred may have been within the period of spontaneous recovery. Another difference, which may be important in understanding the possibilities for rehabilitation of category-specific impairments, is the aetiology of the damage.

The two cases described by Hillis and Caramazza (1991), JJ and PS, also showed a substantial improvement in performance when re-tested 13 months post-stroke and post-head injury respectively. Despite this improvement, their performance continued to show the two opposing category-specific effects outlined above.

Laiacona et al. (1997) also carried out a longitudinal study with LF and EA, mentioned above, both of whom had suffered herpes simplex encephalitis. Between one and two years after the first investigation LF had made a good recovery. EA, in contrast, still showed an impairment. Interestingly, LF's improvement was itself category specific. He improved on non-living things (and on higher frequency items) and not on living things. The authors attempt to account for this dissociation in improvement between categories with respect to the lesser degree of correlation between functional and perceptual attributes of living than non-living things (see Chapter 2).

Methodological issues

There are a number of crucial methodological issues that arise when considering past and future studies in this interesting area.

a) Controlling variables

Variables which may underlie apparent category-specific effects, such as familiarity (Funnell and Sheridan, 1992; Stewart et al., 1992), visual complexity (Stewart et al., 1992) and age of acquisition (Howard et al., 1995), must be taken into account in determining the nature of the impairment.

If claims are to be made concerning a category-specific influence on object decision (e.g. Coltheart et al., 1998), it is important to control the degree of perceptual overlap of pairs of items combined to form non-objects in object decision, across the living and non-living categories.

b) Control performance

Not all studies in this area have used data from normal participants, assuming that controls would perform at ceiling. In studies where controls are tested a number of patterns emerge. Normal elderly participants tend to have more difficulty in naming pictures of living things than non-living things (Laiacona et al., 1993; Moss et al., 1997). Under deadline conditions, normal participants make more errors on naming living than non-living things and the errors tend to be spread across more items in the category (Vitcovitch, Humphreys and Lloyd-Jones, 1993). Finally, controls tend to be (non-significantly) poorer with visual attributes of living things than visual attributes of non-living things (naming to definition: Forde at al., 1997) and poorer with perceptual than functional information (also on naming to definition: Gainotti and Silveri, 1996).

The consistency of these patterns across studies suggests that living things (and perhaps their visual attributes in particular) are in some sense 'harder' to process in these tasks. In this case the pattern of performance shown by people with brain damage who have problems with such items may not differ from normal participants whose performance is taken off ceiling; the category-specific effects that are found may represent an amplification of the normal pattern. If a specific problem with visual features of living things reflects an extreme version of normal performance, it may be that we shall learn most about semantic organization and its breakdown by working with people with the reverse pattern, worse performance on non-living items.

In further work with people with category-specific impairments, of whatever type, it is important to use materials matched for normal performance across categories and attributes. Where normal participants are at ceiling for accuracy, studies with reaction times are crucial in ensuring that sets of stimuli are truly matched for difficulty.

c) Good comprehension

Comprehension tasks that are not performed at ceiling level (e.g. picture name verification, reaction time tasks) are necessary before authors claim category-specific deficits specific to output (see descriptions of studies by Hart et al., 1985 and Farah and Wallace, 1992).

d) Consistency of interpretation

In addition to performing well designed and controlled tasks with people with category-specific disorders, it is essential to interpret scores consistently. A particular example of inconsistency of interpretation is of the results of the object decision task. SE (Moss et al., 1997) scored 26/32 on the difficult version of the task from the Birmingham Object Recognition Battery (BORB) (Riddoch and Humphreys, 1993). Performance, within the control range (22–30), was held to be normal. SBR (Forde et al., 1997) scored 27/32 on object decision from the BORB (version unspecified). This score, more than two standard deviations below the mean for the control subjects (mean 29.8, s.d. 1.2), was described as showing some degree of impairment. Forde et al., (1997) go on to claim that SBR has a general deficit in (a non-categorical) structural descriptions system; this claim is also on the basis of a residual deficit shown in reaction times on object decision when SBR appeared to have recovered.

This inconsistency was revealed by careful cross-study comparison and was clear only because the different researchers used versions of the same task. As this area develops, sensible cross-case comparisons will be possible only where the same results are interpreted in the same way!

e) Testing across modalities of input

The majority of studies assess performance with tasks using words and pictures. While the results can be informative, interpretation may be hampered because of the potential influence of the modality of input on semantic processing. The pattern of performance across a variety of modalities of input (e.g. including testing involving characteristic sounds, touch and even taste) will help clarify the nature of the deficit and should therefore help refine models of processing.

f) Attribute testing to avoid priming

It is not appropriate to probe attribute knowledge by providing several questions about each item together or even on the same occasion of testing. This approach ignores the literature on priming in normals and people with brain damage. The results from online studies should not be ignored in offline testing. The research so far ignores the possibility that earlier questions (e.g. from Laiacona et al., 1993: 'Bicycle – does it have wheels, skates or a propeller?') may provide semantic information that could be used (automatically or strategically) to inform (correctly or incorrectly) the answers to later questions (e.g. 'Bicycle: does it run on pedals, electricity or fuel?'). Ideas from connectionist models (see Chapter 2) are also relevant here. In some models, if the activation of semantic knowledge goes beyond a 'critical mass' then 'pattern completion' may occur: a mild deficit in knowledge of visual attributes, for example, may be obscured if the concept as a whole is activated on the basis of intact associative knowledge. This may be particularly likely if this knowledge has just been primed.

As research begins to include more assessments of attribute knowledge, it is important to probe only one attribute per item on each occasion. If questions about an item have to be blocked, or included in a single session due to time constraints, questions on different attribute types should at least be counterbalanced across items.

Finally, researchers should distinguish between shared and distinctive attributes as these may be differentially impaired (Caramazza and Shelton, 1998; Moss et al., 1997).

Conclusion

In summary, a variety of single cases with deficits restricted by semantic category have been described. While the patterns of disorder do have the potential to inform models of normal processing, several of the case studies are flawed. For example, some have not controlled adequately for variables that have since been shown to be crucial (for a discussion see Funnell and Sheridan, 1992) while others claim category-specific effects in output without comparing across categories on comprehension tasks where performance has been taken 'off ceiling' (e.g. Hart et al. 1985).

The interest in category-specific disorders

> has led to a voluminous literature documenting various patterns of selective semantic impairment. It has not, however, led to any agreement concerning what these patterns of impairment tell us about the nature of semantic memory.
>
> Coltheart et al., 1998: 353–54

This is a rather negative but accurate view. However, two factors from the recent literature can provide us with hope that progress is being made. Firstly, different theories of semantic memory are being elaborated and links made with other areas of research (e.g. concept development, Caramazza and Shelton, 1998; connectionist modelling, Farah and McClelland, 1991; brain imaging, Lambon Ralph et al., 1998). As theories are formed and further specified, so further predictions can be made and tested. Theoretical progress may in fact have been hampered due to the strong appeal of the sensory functional theory and variants thereof (e.g. Farah and McClelland, 1991; Warrington and Shallice, 1984; see Saffran and Schwartz, 1994, for a review of the literature in support of this account). It is only as evidence against this position accumulates that new and modified theories of how our conceptual knowledge is organized begin to emerge.

Secondly, more thorough investigations with people with category-specific impairments are being described. As these incorporate cross-case comparisons (e.g. Lambon Ralph et al., 1998), online tasks (Moss et al.,

1997) and well controlled investigations of attribute knowledge (Laiacona et al., 1993) firmer conclusions can be drawn. However, the methodological issues raised here may also be important in making future progress and in preventing trips down blind alleys.

Research on the rehabilitation of such deficits must also be a priority. As well as having the potential to help some individuals with these impairments, such research also has the potential to inform theory. For example, FM and RG (Laiacona et al., 1993) were impaired on attribute judgements, but only for living things. If it were possible to improve their knowledge of visual properties of living things would this generalize to improved knowledge of functional attributes of living things? Might generalization vary according to how correlated form and function are for particular items?

This chapter will hopefully perform at least two functions. Firstly, that readers, confused about the nature of semantic knowledge, will understand that this is the nature of this area of research: there is no single model that accounts for all neuropsychological data. The topic is confusing but nevertheless both important and interesting. Secondly, the chapter aims to inspire well controlled investigations of people's semantic knowledge after damage and also, where appropriate, to encourage clinicians to carry out treatment studies with people with category-specific deficits.

References

Allport DA (1985) Distributed memory, modular subsystems and dysphasia. In Newman SK, Epstein R, (Eds) Current Perspectives in Dysphasia. Edinburgh: Churchill Livingstone. pp 32–60.

Best W, Nickels L (2000) From theory to therapy in aphasia: where are we now and where to next. Neuropsychological Rehabilitation 10(3): 231–247.

Caramazza A (1998) The interpretation of semantic category specific deficits: what do they reveal about the organization of conceptual knowledge in the brain? Neurocase 4: 265–72.

Caramazza A, Shelton J (1998) Domain specific knowledge systems in the brain: the animate–inanimate distinction. Journal of Cognitive Neuroscience 10: 1–34.

Coltheart M, Inglis L, Cupples L, Michie P, Bates A, Budd B (1998) A semantic subsystem of visual attributes. Neurocase 4: 353–70.

Damasio H, Grabowski TJ, Tranel D, Hichwa RD, Damasio AR (1996) A neural basis for lexical retrieval. Nature 380: 499–505.

De Renzi E, Luchelli F (1994) Are semantic systems separately represented in the brain? The case of living category impairment. Cortex 30: 3–25.

Farah MJ and McClelland JL (1991) A computational model of semantic memory impairment; modality specificity and emergent category specificity. Journal of Experimental Psychology – General 120: 339–57.

Farah MJ, Wallace MA (1992) Semantically-bounded anomia; implications for the neural implementation of naming. Neuropsychologia 30: 609–21.

Forde EME, Francis D, Riddoch MJ, Rumiati RI, Humphreys GW (1997) On the links between visual knowledge and naming: a single case study of a patient with a category specific impairment for living things. Cognitive Neuropsychology 14: 403–58.

Funnell E, De Mornay Davies P (1996) JBR: a reassessment of concept familiarity and a category specific disorder for living things. Neurocase 2: 461–74.

Funnell E, Sheridan J (1992) Categories of knowledge? Unfamiliar aspects of living and non-living things. Cognitive Neuropsychology 9: 135–53.

Gainotti G, Silveri MC (1996) Cognitive and anatomical locus of lesion in a patient with a category specific semantic impairment for living things. Cognitive Neuropsychology 13: 357–89.

Gonnerman LM, Andersen ES, Devlin JT, Kemplar D, Seidenberg MS (1997) Double dissociation of semantic categories in Alzheimer's disease. Brain and Language 57: 254–79.

Hart J, Berndt RS, Caramazza A (1985) Category specific naming deficit following cerebral infarction. Nature 316: 439–40.

Hillis AE, Caramazza A (1991) Category specific naming and comprehension impairment: a double dissociation. Brain 114: 2081–94.

Howard D, Best W, Bruce C, Gatehouse C (1995) Operativity and animacy effects in aphasic naming. Special issue in honour of Ruth Lesser. European Journal of Disorders of Communication 30: 286–302.

Howard D, Orchard-Lisle VM (1984) On the origin of semantic errors in naming: evidence from the case of a global aphasic. Cognitive Neuropsychology 1: 163–90.

Humphreys GW, Riddoch MJ, Quinlan P (1988) Cascade processes in picture identification. Cognitive Neuropsychology 5: 67–103.

Laiacona M, Barbarotto R, Capitani E (1993) Perceptual and associative knowledge in category specific impairment of semantic memory: a study of two cases. Cortex 29: 727–40.

Laiacona M, Capitani E, Barbarotto R(1997) Semantic category dissociations: a longitudinal study of two cases. Cortex 33: 441–61.

Lambon Ralph MA, Howard D, Nightingale G, Ellis AW (1998) Are living and non-living category specific deficits causally linked to impaired perceptual or associative knowledge? Evidence from a category specific double dissociation. Neurocase 4: 311–38.

Laws KR, Evans JJ, Hodges JR, McCarthy RA (1995) Naming without knowing and appearance without associations: evidence for constructive processes in semantic memory? Memory 3: 409–33.

McCarthy RA, Warrington EK (1988) Evidence for modality-specific meaning systems in the brain. Nature 334: 428–30.

Moss HE, Tyler LK, Jennings F (1997) When leopards lose their spots: knowledge of visual properties in category specific deficits for living things. Cognitive Neuropsychology 14: 901–50.

Riddoch MJ, Humphreys GW (1993) BORB: Birmingham Object Recognition Battery. Hove: Lawrence Erlbaum Associates Ltd.

Sacchett C, Humphreys GW (1992) Calling a squirrel a squirrel, but a canoe a wigwam: a category specific deficit for artefactual objects and body parts. Cognitive Neuropsychology 9: 73–86.

Saffran EM, Schwartz MF (1994) Of cabbages and things; semantic memory from a neuropsychological perspective – a tutorial review. In Umilta C, Moscovitch M, (Eds)

Attention and Performance 15: Conscious and nonconscious information processing. Cambridge MA: MIT Press. pp 507–36.

Sartori G, Job R (1988) The oyster with four legs: a neuropsychological study on the interaction of visual and semantic information. Cognitive Neuropsychology 5: 105–32.

Sartori G, Miozzo M, Job R (1994) Rehabilitation of semantic memory impairments. In Riddoch MJ, Humphreys GW, (Eds) Cognitive neuropsychology and cognitive rehabilitation. Hove: Lawrence Erlbaum Associates.

Shallice T (1988) From Neuropsychology to Mental Structure. Cambridge; Cambridge University Press.

Sheridan J, Humphreys GW (1993) A verbal-semantic category specific recognition impairment. Cognitive Neuropsychology 10: 143–84.

Silveri MC, Gainotti G (1988) Interaction between vision and language in category specific semantic impairment. Cognitive Neuropsychology 5: 677–709.

Snodgrass JG, Vanderwart M (1980) A standardised set of 260 pictures: norms for name agreement, familiarity, and visual complexity. Journal of Experimental Psychology – General 6: 174–215.

Stewart F, Parkin AJ, Hunkin NM (1992) Naming impairment following recovery from herpes simplex encephalitis: category specific? Quarterly Journal of Experimental Psychology 44A: 261–84.

Swales M, Johnson R (1992) Patients with semantic memory loss: can they relearn lost concepts? Neuropsychological Rehabilitation 2: 295–305.

Vitcovitch M, Humphreys GW, Loyd-Jones TJ (1993) Perseverative responding in speeded naming to pictures: it's in the links. Journal of Experimental Psychology: Learning, Memory and Cognition 17: 664–80.

Warrington EK (1975) The selective impairment of semantic memory. Quarterly Journal of Experimental Psychology 27: 635–57.

Warrington EK, Shallice T (1984) Category specific semantic impairment. Brain 107: 829–54.

Warrington EK and McCarthy RA (1987) Categories of knowledge: further fractionations and an attempted integration. Brain 110: 1273–96.

CHAPTER 5

Semantics and therapy in aphasia

Lyndsey Nickels

Introduction

We all have a store of the meanings of words that we know. This store is commonly referred to as the semantic system and is essential for both understanding and producing language. In order that we can understand what is said to us we have to refer to the stored meanings of each word and, similarly, when we want to express an idea we select the word with the appropriate meaning for that idea. Thus, semantics plays a central role in language, mediating in all forms of language understanding and expression, both spoken and written.

Disorders of semantics are a common feature of aphasia. The fact that semantic processing is an essential component for communication – involved in both language comprehension and production – makes it a key cause for concern and often a priority for remediation. Because of this critical role, much time in clinical practice is justifiably devoted to attempting to improve semantic processing in order to effect an improvement in the comprehension and production of the person with aphasia. Here, we shall concentrate on the findings from research and discuss what they can illuminate at the present time regarding effective treatment in this complex area.

Semantic therapy or therapy for semantics?

It is important to draw a distinction between the nature of the task used for remediation and the nature of the deficit that is to be remediated. Many if not all tasks involve semantic processing because of its pivotal role in language and communication. However, there are clearly some tasks which are explicitly designed to focus on semantic processing, while others focus on different processing components (e.g. 'minimal pairs' tasks aim to focus on early auditory analysis). Examples of 'semantic' tasks that are commonly used in the clinical setting are 'odd one out', and picture or object selection from an array.

The former usually involves presentation of three or more words, pictures or objects where all but one are selected from the same semantic category (e.g. cat, dog, rabbit, house). The object of the task is to correctly identify the object that is from a different semantic category. The task can be graded in difficulty, with the aim of increasing the specificity of semantic processing required. For example, 'house' could be replaced with 'lion' so that the difference between the 'odd-one-out' and distractors is reduced.

It is by no means certain, however, that this assumption of graded difficulty is valid for all aphasic people. As is discussed later in this paper, Morris (1997) found that rated semantic similarity of target and distractor affected performance of only one of two aphasics on a word–picture verification task. Moreover, in studies of the facilitation of aphasic naming no effect has been found on the 'depth of semantic processing' – which equates to the 'closeness' of semantic distractors (Barry and McHattie, 1991; Howard, Patterson, Franklin et al., 1985a).

As with the 'odd-one-out' task, the selection task involves presentation of several pictures or objects, and the person with aphasia is required to select the item named by the clinician. The 'difficulty' of the task or of the semantic processing involved is altered by manipulating the relationship of the items in the array: they may be unrelated items from a range of semantic categories (e.g. dog, house, car, tree), or closely related items from one semantic category (e.g. dog, cat, rabbit, mouse), or, of course, somewhere between the two, using items from wider superordinate categories (e.g. dog, lion, shark, eagle).

While it is clear that these tasks all involve semantic processing and are explicitly designed to do so, this does not necessarily mean that they will be used to improve or will result in an improvement in semantic processing. Indeed, tasks just like these have been used in published therapy studies where no mention has been made of their effects on impairments of semantic processing (e.g. Davis and Pring, 1991; Howard, Patterson, Franklin et al., 1985b). Many of these studies describe their therapy as 'semantic therapy' because at their core is the use of tasks that rely on semantic processing for their successful completion (e.g. Nickels and Best, 1996a, 1996b). However, this is different from the claim that the aim of the therapy is to remediate semantics – indeed, the majority of the recent studies that involve 'semantic therapy' aim to improve word finding (usually measured using picture naming) rather than semantic processing itself.

We shall divide our discussion of the remediation of semantic processing into three parts. First, we shall discuss the use of semantic tasks in the remediation of word finding – suggesting that for some people with aphasia these tasks are indeed acting at the level of semantic processing but that for others this may not be the case. Next, we shall discuss other studies where tasks that do not explicitly focus on semantic processing do seem to produce results that suggest a semantic locus for the effects of therapy. Finally, we shall turn to those studies that focus more explicitly on remediation of semantic processing (or therapy for semantics) including assessment of both comprehension and production.

Semantic tasks in the facilitation of word finding

'Semantic' tasks such as word–picture matching are now widely used in the remediation of disorders of word finding, and in the majority of studies reported these tasks do improve the picture naming of the person with aphasia with whom they have been used (Nickels and Best, 1996a, 1996b). However, it is not the case that this improvement is always attributed to improved semantic processing. For example, Marshall, Pound, White-Thompson et al. (1990) suggest that following treatment using written word–picture matching (with semantically related distractors) the improvement of one man's anomia was due to a strengthening of the links between the semantic and phonological levels of processing. This section considers treatment studies that give us insights into how semantically based tasks may be influencing processing, noting that tasks may achieve their effects in different ways for different people.

While Marshall et al. argued against the effects of treatment occurring at a semantic level, some authors have suggested that in other aphasic people the same task does facilitate naming by acting at the level of the (impaired) semantic system. For example, Hillis and Caramazza (1994) describe JJ, a person with aphasia, who was identified as having a semantic deficit – he made semantic errors on both written and spoken naming and word–picture matching. To improve JJ's spoken naming they used a task involving selection of the appropriate picture (from an array of 40) to match a written word, giving him feedback regarding accuracy and correcting incorrect responses. JJ showed significant improvement on subsequent naming of the treated items. In contrast, he showed no improvement in naming when treated using phonemic cues to elicit a correct reading response for the names of the pictures (without the picture being present). Hillis and Caramazza propose that the semantically based therapy was effective because JJ's deficit was at the level of the semantic system. They suggest that perhaps the therapy had facilitated naming by teaching distinctions between or by activating features that distinguish semantically related items. If indeed this was the case then improvement should have been predicted on written naming and comprehension of the same items. In particular, accuracy on the word–picture matching task should have improved during the course of therapy, but unfortunately this was not discussed.

One of the most interesting findings from these studies is that semantic tasks (usually word–picture matching) can still have an effect on a person's word production even when their semantic processing is good enough to perform the task accurately. For example, TRC (Nickels and Best, 1996b) scored 97% correct on matching a written word to one of four pictures (with semantically related distractors) during therapy, and yet showed a significant and lasting improvement in his naming of the treated items after therapy finished. This makes it seem unlikely that for TRC the therapy had been effective by teaching distinctions between semantically related items (as argued by Hillis and Caramazza, 1994, for JJ). As he can do the word–picture matching task (where distractors are semantically related), it seems that he already 'knows' the distinctions between these items. Yet, Nickels and Best (1996b) do argue that the source of TRC's improved naming is at the level of semantics, because he showed improved written naming of the treated items as well as improved spoken naming. The equivalent improvement in both written and spoken modalities implicates a common level of processing (i.e. semantics) as the source of this improvement.

However, it is not necessarily the case that accuracy on the task implies intact semantic processing: certainly, on other assessments of semantics (such as synonym judgements) TRC showed evidence of impairment. Clearly, then, there are two possibilities regarding the effects of therapy on TRC's semantic processing more generally – either it was improved or it was not! TRC's improvement, although in both spoken and written naming, was primarily restricted to those items treated in therapy (with a transient improvement on untreated items that lasted less than one month). This would appear to suggest not that a general improvement in the functioning of the semantic system had occurred but rather that there had been some item-specific facilitation for the treated items (which may have been at the level of semantics).

It is clear that improved naming can be achieved using semantic tasks even in aphasic people who appear to have good semantic processing. For at least some of these people the source of the improvement seems most likely to be at the level of the semantic system. This leads to two hypotheses regarding the mechanism for this improvement:

1. Although performance on tests of (input) semantics appears good, it may be that our tests just aren't sensitive enough. Thus, although semantic processing is sufficient to succeed on a forced-choice comprehension task, it is not sufficient to support naming. It would follow then that the semantic processing involved in this task can help clarify semantic distinctions to support word output, even for aphasic people like TRC who can perform word–picture matching accurately.

2. The second possibility is that, indeed, semantic processing is intact – at least for the concrete items used in the picture-naming task – but repeated semantic activation of a particular item still facilitates naming. Jones (1989) suggested that performing a semantic task could provide more 'semantic drive' to overcome a subsequent problem in activation of the lexical representation for output. That is to say, there is (long-term) semantic priming for a particular item, as a result of performing the semantic task. This higher level of activation of the primed item will in turn lead to more activation addressing the lexical representation, which – in a damaged system – may increase the chance of successful retrieval.

Both of these accounts predict improvement restricted to those stimuli used in therapy – and in the vast majority of cases reported this is exactly what has been found (e.g. Marshall et al., 1990). However, it is not entirely clear whether either or both of these accounts might also predict improved input processing for those items (i.e. speed and/or accuracy of access for comprehension). Unfortunately, the appropriate testing of comprehension has not been carried out in most studies.

So, while semantic tasks can be effective at remediating word finding, it may not be that in every case it is by acting at the level of semantics. For some people the task might result in better 'links' between semantics and phonology and for others an effect at the level of phonology (e.g. lowering the threshold of an output phonological representation by repeated use). Thus, very often the precise mechanism by which these tasks are effective is not clear for a particular person and more research is clearly needed. Nevertheless word–picture matching is clearly a useful task, and has been shown to be effective at remediating word finding with many different people with anomia, of differing strengths and deficits in language processing. Before turning our attention to studies that have more explicitly focused on remediating semantic deficits, we shall discuss a study that uses a task that would not generally be classified as overtly semantic but yet appears to have resulted in improved semantic processing.

Remediation of semantic deficits without the use of explicitly semantic tasks?

Hillis (1989; patient 1) used a cueing hierarchy to remediate the written naming of a man with aphasia, who had a semantic deficit. The cueing hierarchy involved progressive cues to assist production of the written name. Initially, a picture was presented, and he was encouraged to write the name of the picture. If he was unable to do so, a scrambled anagram was given, initially with two extra distractor letters, then without distractor letters. If naming was still not achieved, this was followed by an initial letter cue, then by the spoken name – for writing to dictation – and finally by brief presentation of the written name for delayed copying. Hillis reports that following around six sessions of treatment using the hierarchy, there was improved writing of the treated items and also improvement on spoken naming of the same items, and on spoken and written naming of untreated items in the same semantic category. This improvement was maintained for around 20 sessions after therapy had been discontinued.

The fact that both spoken and written naming benefited from therapy for this man who had a semantic deficit suggests that the therapy had effected an improvement in semantic processing, and yet the therapy task is not one that would be immediately considered as being primarily semantic in its focus. Clearly, as picture naming is the goal, semantic activation must occur during the processing of the picture and attempts to name the picture, but the nature of the cues place the focus firmly on orthographic information when naming is unsuccessful. However, this may be misleading: although the route to provision of the target is via ortho-graphic, and then phonological, cues, it may be the provision of the target itself that is critical. In other words, for this man who made semantic errors in naming, it may have been the fact that he was always given the correct response that effected the improvement in semantic processing, *not* the process by which this response was achieved. The feedback on the nature of his initial naming response – predominantly semantic errors – and provi-sion or generation of the correct response may be the critical elements of the treatment for this man. This process would allow him to reflect on the distinctions (in meaning) between his response and the target. Thus, it is possible that an amended form of the therapy where this man was told whether his attempt at naming the picture was correct and then provided, if necessary, with the target would have been equally successful.

This study emphasizes the complexities of interpreting the interactions between task, deficit and outcome. Clearly a superficial consideration of task requirements may be misleading since, although this was an orthographic cueing hierarchy, what seems plausible is that the important element was the opportunity to reflect on differences between targets and semantically related errors.

Semantic tasks in the remediation of semantic deficits

We now turn to look at studies that have set out more explicitly to remediate semantic processing, as opposed to the studies discussed above that have aimed primarily to remediate naming, even though this may have been achieved by improved semantic processing. The first factor that becomes apparent is that there is a relative lack of published reports of studies in this area. More specifically, despite the importance of remediation of semantic processing for the person with aphasia, and thus for the clinician involved in their management, there are few published reports that use a single case study design with suitable controls that enable evaluation of the efficacy of therapy. The main features of six studies – presented in chronological order – are outlined below, as a sample that illustrates different types of therapy and different outcomes.

1. Scott (1987)

This study describes a remediation programme for an aphasic man, AB, who was impaired in all aspects of language requiring semantic mediation as a result of a central semantic processing deficit. The aim of the programme was to improve his semantic processing abilities by enabling access to more precise levels of semantic information about words and pictures. Therapy was carried out using pictures and the auditory input modality alone, for three times a week over three months. The emphasis throughout was on comprehension rather than expression, and therapy comprised a range of tasks, all of which were considered to require a degree of semantic processing. The tasks were graded so that they became increasingly difficult and demanded 'finer' semantic judgements. Included in the tasks were the following: gross and fine picture and word categorization/classification; 'odd-one-out' with increasingly fine distinctions; word (and definition) to picture matching with semantic distractors; word–picture verification tasks; and yes/no statements. Unfortunately AB had a second cerebrovascular accident 11 weeks into the 12-week programme. Nevertheless, he significantly improved on a range of auditory and picture comprehension tasks, and on naming treated and untreated items, with no improvement on control tasks. However, there was no generalization to written comprehension tasks as might have been expected from a change in central semantic processes.

2. Byng (1988); Byng and Coltheart (1986)

BRB, a man with aphasia, was given therapy focusing on his poor comprehension of abstract words. Two different treatment tasks were used sequentially. The first was a picture–word matching task, in which BRB was required to perceive relationships between pictures representing abstract words and the meaning of the word: he was given sheets consisting of the written word plus four pictures on a page – taken from the Shallice and McGill (unpublished) word–picture matching test – and was instructed to select the picture he thought went best with the word. Having completed the set he then checked his responses against a list of answers. The therapy produced treated-item-specific results which generalized from the written word–picture matching therapy to auditory word–picture matching in testing. However, these results were task specific – that is, there was improved comprehension only on the treated word–picture matching task and no carry-over to a synonym judgement task. This task-specific improvement suggests, at best, only a limited, and possibly erroneous, understanding of each word's meaning based on the picture, and, at worst, merely a paired-associate learning of which picture went with which word.

The second task required BRB to generate one-word synonyms for a set of abstract words, which requires quite careful thought about the shades of meaning within words. In order to do this BRB had to consult a diction-ary, look at the different meanings for each word and make up his own synonym that best encapsulated the range of meanings. After four weeks of this regime there was significant improvement in his abstract word comprehension. Once again, the effects were item specific, but here there was carry-over to another task – picture–word matching with the synonyms of the treated items. This suggests that this dictionary therapy could prove to be a useful method of improving comprehension of a specific set of words but that the improvement may not generalize to untreated words.

3. Behrmann and Lieberthal (1989)

This study aimed to improve the comprehension of single items in a globally aphasic man, CH. He was demonstrated to have a severe comprehension deficit irrespective of modality of input. Behrmann and Lieberthal suggest that CH had a central semantic deficit – specifically an inability to obtain a precise semantic specification of an item. The remediation programme used a category-specific approach to assess whether improvement that might be obtained on item-specific training might generalize within and across categories. The therapy tasks (in 15 sessions over six weeks) comprised two major stages. The first was aimed at teaching meaning at a general level of description, i.e. teaching the superordinate features of each category (similarity of group identity). The second was aimed at teaching specific details (or semantic features) of items leading to the precise identification of these items (selection to definition with increasingly close semantic distractors).

Following therapy, CH showed a significant improvement in comprehension of treated items in all the three treated categories (as measured by a categorization task). Overall there was a significant improvement in the untreated items in the treated categories and no improvement in the untreated categories. However, while the overall effects are as described, within the treated categories only one category showed a marked improvement on untreated items, and within the untreated categories marked improvement was also shown for one category. Nevertheless, the therapy was effective and significant improvements were also obtained on other measures of comprehension.

4. Hillis (1990)

Hillis reports a therapy study carried out with a woman with aphasia, HG, who produced comparable types and rates of semantic errors in a number of different tasks (oral and written naming, repetition, writing to dictation, and auditory and written word–picture matching). This pattern suggested a deficit at the level of the semantic system. Hillis hypothesized that the semantic impairment entailed degraded distinctions between related words. For example, HG produced 'lion' when naming a picture of a tiger. Hillis suggests that an impoverished semantic representation of 'tiger' (identifying it merely as a feline, or large, wild feline) could activate output representations for both tiger and lion. She therefore used a treatment that was designed to re-teach distinctions between semantically related items. HG was required to attempt to name a picture – if she produced a semantic error then the referent of this response was drawn and the contrasting semantic features between her response and the target were identified. Hillis gives the example of HG producing 'lemon' in response to a picture of a cherry. In this case the clinician drew a lemon and pointed out the differences between a cherry and a lemon (yellow/red, elliptical/ round, sour/sweet, tough/tender skin, etc.). After around twelve therapy sessions, written naming of the treated items had reached ceiling and this semantic therapy was stopped. HG showed generalization of improvement to comprehension (auditory word–picture matching), oral naming, repetition and writing to dictation for these same items. There was also generalization to untreated items that belonged to the same semantic category as the treated words – naming was both more accurate and fewer semantic errors were produced on both naming and in word–picture matching. However, there was no improvement on untreated items from different semantic categories.

Hillis suggests that the most probable mechanism for improvements associated with the semantic treatment was that teaching semantic distinctions between trained items and related items resulted in relearning of, or improved access to, semantic information. Thus, learning these distinctions might (and, for HG, did) increase the probability of producing trained words as correct responses and reduce the probability of producing trained words as error responses to untrained related stimuli. In other words, to use the example above, the therapy would result in improved naming of both the treated item 'cherry' and also the semantically related item 'lemon' that appeared in therapy. In one sense, then, at least some of the so-called 'untreated' semantically related items were actually treated, as presumably they were discussed during the therapy. One wonders whether there was a difference in outcome between untreated items that had and had not appeared during therapy.

5. Grayson, Hilton and Franklin (1997)

This study reports a series of therapies carried out within the first six months post-onset in the treatment of LR, a man with dysphasia. LR was demonstrated to have a profound semantic deficit and additional auditory processing impairments. The initial phase of therapy concentrated on semantic processing using three different tasks.

1. *Spoken and/or written word–object/picture matching.* Task complexity was slowly increased by adding more distractors (starting with one) and by moving from unrelated to related distractors. Additional cues were given to assist LR in his response if necessary, including gesture and provision of additional semantic information.
2. *Categorization.* This also used a multi-modality approach, provided additional cues where necessary, and increased task complexity (how similar the categories were) over time.
3. *Matching associates.* (e.g. carpenter–saw, painter–brush).

Following this therapy, LR showed improved performance on both written and spoken word–picture matching (where the stimuli had not been treated), with fewer errors where unrelated distractors were selected. There was no change on an auditory discrimination task or sentence–picture matching during this phase of therapy, but, in a crossover design, each of these tasks improved when therapy was directed at the appropriate level of processing. Spontaneous speech was also seen to improve during the course of therapy but, as the authors acknowledge, they were unable to attribute this unambiguously to the effects of therapy.

6. Morris (1997)

Morris used the same therapy technique with two different people with aphasia, AD and JAC, both of whom were identified as having semantic deficits with difficulties on tasks involving access to semantics across all presentation modalities. The therapy involved the use of a spoken word–picture verification task: a picture was presented together with either the correct name or a semantically related name (orally presented), and a decision made whether the name should be accepted or rejected as the name of the picture. For example, a picture of a lion would be shown with either the word *lion* or *tiger*. AD and JAC were given immediate feedback regarding the accuracy of their decision. If they were incorrect, they were given both the correct and the semantically related word in written form, and required to point to which was the correct name (both AD and JAC tended to show better comprehension of written material). If an incorrect choice was made brief oral descriptions were given regarding the similarities and differences between the target and semantic distractor. Neither JAC nor AD was required to produce any spoken output during the therapy sessions. JAC received twelve 30–40 minute sessions of therapy (two/three sessions a week). AD received nine longer sessions, seeing each treatment picture twice rather than once, as was the case for JAC.

Following therapy, JAC and AD were reassessed on the spoken word–picture verification task, involving both treated and untreated items. JAC had improved significantly on both treated and untreated items; moreover he also showed improvement on some related semantic tasks, such as the Pyramids and Palm Trees test (Howard and Patterson, 1992: one spoken word – two written word version). No change was observed on control tasks (word reading) nor on a written word–picture verification task or written picture naming, and prior to therapy JAC had shown stable baselines, suggesting that these improvements were indeed the result of therapy. Much of the observed improvement was maintained when JAC was reassessed four months later. Morris suggests that the therapy is unlikely to have been effective by improving semantic information itself (supported by the lack of improvement on picture naming and the written version of the word–picture verification task). She argues instead that the improvement results from improved access to semantic information from the auditory modality alone.

In contrast to JAC, AD failed to show any significant change following therapy, either on the treated task or on related semantic tasks. He did show improved spoken picture naming but only if self-corrected responses were included. AD was subsequently given a further period of therapy with amended feedback to ensure comprehension. Instead of just being given the written names he was also given the picture of the semantically related distractor. Following this phase of therapy AD did show improved performance on the word–picture verification task, but this was restricted to treated items. There was no generalization of performance to untreated items nor to any other semantic tasks or picture naming.

Discussion: The remediation of semantic deficits

The studies described above all involved people with aphasia who had impairments at the level of semantics. All of the studies set out to remediate these deficits using tasks that are part of the standard therapeutic repertoire of the speech and language therapist. The studies use pre- and post-therapy measures combined with control tasks to determine the efficacy of the therapy, and examine generalization across items, tasks and modalities. Overall it can be said that the outcome of the studies is very positive – all the studies show that the therapy resulted in some degree of improvement and many demonstrate generalization of some kind. However, it is clear that the studies do differ in the type and extent of generalization. Thus, some of the therapy studies resulted in item-specific improvement (Byng, 1988) or modality-specific improvement (Morris, 1997: JAC), while others show generalization across items (Morris, 1997: JAC) and/or across modalities (Hillis, 1990). The different patterns of generalization are generally used to infer the locus of the effects of therapy within the language processing system. For example, Morris (1997) argues for an improvement of access to semantic information from the auditory modality alone to account for the generalization to untreated items but not to untreated modalities (written comprehension, spoken or written output) for JAC.

What is apparent is that despite the fact that all these studies used semantic tasks with people who had central semantic deficits, with the aim of remediating these deficits, they did not all produce the same outcome. Before discussing some of the possible factors that may underlie these differences, I should like to note the common theme that is emerging from recent research in aphasia therapy. Simply put, it is that the results of therapy are complex and difficult to interpret, and even more difficult to predict. I do not intend to discuss this issue in depth here, but urge that this complexity should be interpreted as being a natural point in the evolution of this area of research. We have established that many different types of therapy are effective for many different people with different language deficits, and the next logical step is to refine our understanding of which therapy is effective for which problem – with the ultimate goal of being able to predict accurately the outcome of therapy. In order to be able to do this successfully, we need to identify the precise demands of a therapy task and examine in detail (at a level hitherto rarely attempted) how they interact with the aphasic person's areas of deficit and areas of strength. These issues are discussed further by Best and Nickels (2000) and Nickels and Best (1996a, 1996b).

With respect to the possible factors that may underlie differences in the effects of therapy across the studies described above, there are two obvious sources of these factors: differences between participants and differences between therapy tasks. The discussion will now focus on these two factors.

Differences between participants

The people with aphasia described here were argued to have 'central semantic deficits' with resulting impairments in all modalities of input and output. In this sense they could be said to be similar – however, they undoubtedly had different co-occurring deficits which could affect their response to therapy.

For example, in discussing the different responses of JAC and AD to the same therapy procedure, Morris (1997) suggests that differences in their naming ability may have played a role. JAC was able to benefit from the therapy when feedback involved written words and verbal explanation, whereas AD, who had very similar auditory comprehension skills to JAC, required pictorial cues as feedback to enable him to benefit. Morris suggests that JAC's superior naming abilities might have enabled him to generate – sometimes – the name of the picture prior to hearing the target or distractor name in the word–picture verification task, which could assist his judgement of the stimulus word. This account, she argues, is supported by the increase in JAC's false positive responses following therapy. In contrast, AD's naming was slow, laborious and rarely correct and it is unlikely therefore that he would have been able to generate the target name to assist in his processing of the spoken word.

In addition to differences in the pattern of co-occurring deficits, it is also more than likely that our analysis of the semantic disorder itself is insufficiently detailed and that not all of these people have identical semantic deficits. Morris (1997), for example, is unusual in examining the factors affecting performance on the word–picture verification task for JAC and AD. In particular, it was found that JAC's performance was predicted by how close the semantic relationship was between the target and the distractor. AD, however, was found not to be affected by this factor. Thus, it seems that the nature of the breakdown in semantic processing may be different for JAC and AD, which could be another plausible source of variance when considering the outcome of therapy.

Semantic disorders can also be distinguished in terms of whether there is a *loss* of stored semantic information (a storage deficit) or whether there is a difficulty in *accessing* information that has remained intact. It is clear that these two different types of semantic breakdown could have different implications for the outcome of therapy.

For example, tasks involving semantic processing could improve the general access procedures in a person where access is impaired but semantic information itself remains intact. This would result in improvement on all tasks involving semantic access and generalization from treated to untreated items. Even where a semantic access deficit does occur, however, there is the possibility that therapy may result in item-specific effects as the result of facilitating access to that particular item alone. This then raises the question of whether such item-specific facilitator effects might also be modality specific. The answer, as so often, must depend on the precise nature of the assumptions made about language processing within the theoretical model being used.

In contrast, if semantic information is lost, item-specific improvement seems the most likely, since information will be 'relearned' regarding specific items, with generalization across tasks and modalities but not from treated to untreated items. Although item-specific effects are certainly the most likely, it is possible that some generalization may occur – particularly within a semantic category. This is likely to depend on the nature of the therapy, but one could imagine the situation where, having relearned that a lion is a wild animal, this is extended to include other (visually) similar animals, for example, tiger and leopard – and possibly extended erroneously to the domestic cat.

Thus, important differences between aphasic people may be of two types: differences in the patterns of strengths and deficits in other language areas that co-occur with their semantic deficit; and differences in the nature of the semantic deficit itself. Either of these two differences could affect the outcome of therapy.

Differences between tasks

There is a striking difference between these studies of therapy for semantic disorders and those studies using 'semantic therapy' for word-finding discussed earlier.

Many of the studies that aimed to remediate semantic processing talk in terms of 're-teaching' distinctions or meanings. It is by no means clear that they are necessarily assuming that there is a loss of semantic information for the aphasics involved. Certainly, the assessments of semantics reported rarely claim to investigate whether an access or storage deficit is implicated. However, they use tasks where feedback is given and differences between correct and incorrect responses are made explicit.

In contrast, in most of the studies using 'semantic therapy' for word-finding, no feedback is given regarding the accuracy of the response, and the emphasis is instead on the facilitatory nature of performing the task. Indeed, as was discussed earlier, many of the people with aphasia perform at ceiling on the tasks. Is the nature of the task important? Unfortunately, to answer this question unequivocally we would need to use both types of task with the same people. For example, would the same pattern of improvement have been shown by HG (Hillis, 1990) if she had been treated using word–picture matching instead of with the naming task with explicit discussion of errors?

Nickels and Best (1996b) report a study that goes some way to answer this question. AER was given two different semantic tasks, both of which improved his picture naming. One was word–picture matching, which produced the effects so often reported – a robust, lasting improvement for naming treated items, together with a transient improvement on untreated items. The other task, 'relatedness judgements', was based on a similar task used by Jones (1989). This involved presentation of a target picture (e.g. cup) with several other pictures, some of which were related in meaning to the target (e.g. plate, drinking, coffee) and some of which were not (e.g. horse, running, paint). AER was required to judge whether each picture was related to the target. In the first phase of therapy, AER performed the task on his own with no feedback. Subsequently the therapy was repeated, but with AER's wife discussing his decisions with him at the end of each session. In contrast to the word–picture matching therapy where AER's performance was close to ceiling, he made a substantial number of errors on this task. The first phase of therapy, with no feedback, resulted in improved naming only for the treated items. However, the second phase, with feedback, resulted in improved naming for both treated and untreated items. Thus, while the 'relatedness judgements' task did result in improved naming, it was only when there was a feedback element incorporated into the task that generalization was obtained. It is also of interest that both the relatedness judgements and word–picture matching resulted in improvement for the treated items, despite the fact that one task was performed much more accurately than the other.

The results of the study with AER suggest that there may be important differences in the effects of a therapy task depending on how the task is presented – in particular, whether or not feedback is given. It is clear, however, that not only the presence or absence of feedback needs to be considered: the exact nature of that feedback can also differ. For example, Hillis (1990) used a contrastive method with HG, explicitly contrasting the features of the target and error, as did Morris (1997). In contrast, Behrmann and Lieberthal (1989) concentrated on the features of the target, selecting the target from distractors on the basis of the features, while Scott (1987) and Grayson et al (1997) didn't explicitly discuss distinctions between stimuli (although, of course, to perform the tasks accurately the stimuli needed to be accurately distinguished). However, while we can see the differences between the nature of the feedback used in the tasks, there is no clear relationship between this and the type and extent of generalization observed in each study. Nevertheless, the type of feedback provided is undoubtedly an important factor. This is particularly clear in the study by Morris (1997) where a change in the nature of the feedback with AD made the difference in the efficacy of the therapy.

Conclusions

A disorder at the level of semantic processing often has a profound and disabling effect on a person's language. It is central to communication whatever its modality (spoken, written, gestural) or combination of modalities. Clearly, the remediation of semantic disorders is a high priority, and what emerges from the literature so far is that semantic tasks are very often effective in therapy. However, the change effected may not always be in the disordered semantic system per se. It may instead be a modality-specific improvement in access to or from that system, for example, in improved spoken naming, or in auditory comprehension. Moreover, the extent of the change, in terms of generalization across items and modalities, can be influenced by the nature of the task and the feedback provided. Clinically, then, it is essential to monitor the efficacy of the therapy task, and to modify that task if the improvement obtained is less than optimal (or, indeed, nonexistent). This should include monitoring of the effects of therapy on treated and untreated items across modalities – auditory and written; comprehension and production. In terms of furthering our understanding of the relationship between task, disorder and outcome, we need to refine our understanding of the nature of semantic breakdown and perform a series of single case therapy studies investigating the effects of identical tasks with different aphasic people, and different tasks with the same people.

Acknowledgements

This paper was written while the author was in receipt of a Fellowship from the Wellcome Trust. Thanks to Wendy Best and Julie Morris for helpful comments on earlier versions of the manuscript.

References

Barry C, McHattie J (1991) Depth of semantic processing in picture naming facilitation in aphasic patients. Paper presented at the British Aphasiology Society Conference, Sheffield: September 1991.

Behrmann M, Lieberthal T (1989) Category-specific treatment of a lexical-semantic deficit: a single case study of global aphasia. British Journal of Disorders of Communication 24: 281–99.

Best WM, Nickels LA (2000) From theory to therapy in aphasia: where are we now and where to next? Neuropsychological Rehabilitation 10(3): 231–47.

Byng S (1988) Sentence processing deficits: theory and therapy. Cognitive Neuropsychology 5: 629–76.

Byng S, Coltheart M (1986) Aphasia therapy research: methodological requirements and illustrative results. In Hjelmquist E, Nilsson L-G, (Eds) Communication and Handicap: Aspects of Psychological Compensation and Technical Aids. New York: North Holland Elsevier Science.

Davis A, Pring T (1991) Therapy for word finding deficits: more on the effects of semantic and phonological approaches to treatment with dysphasic patients. Neuropsychological Rehabilitation: 135–45.

Grayson E, Hilton R, Franklin SE (1997) Early intervention in a case of jargon aphasia: efficacy of language comprehension therapy. European Journal of Disorders of Communication 32: 257–76.

Hillis AE (1989) Efficacy and generalization of treatment for aphasic naming errors. Archives of Physical Medicine Rehabilitation 70: 632–36.

Hillis AE (1990) Effects of separate treatments for distinct impairments within the naming process. In Prescott T, (Ed) Clinical Aphasiology: 19. Austin, TA: Pro-Ed. pp 255–65.

Hillis A, Caramazza A (1994) Theories of lexical processing and rehabilitation of lexical deficits. In Riddoch MJ, Humphreys GW, (Eds) Cognitive Neuropsychology and Cognitive Rehabilitation. Hove: Lawrence Erlbaum Associates.

Howard D, Patterson KE (1992) The Pyramids and Palm Trees Test. Bury St Edmunds: Thames Valley Test Company.

Howard D, Patterson KE, Franklin S, Orchard-Lisle V, Morton J (1985a) The facilitation of picture naming in aphasia. Cognitive Neuropsychology 2: 49–80.

Howard D, Patterson KE, Franklin S, Orchard-Lisle V, Morton J (1985b) The treatment of word retrieval deficits in aphasia: a comparison of two therapy methods. Brain 108: 817–29.

Jones EV (1989) A year in the life of EVJ and PC. Proceedings of the Summer Conference of the British Aphasiology Society, June 1989: Cambridge.

Marshall J, Pound C, White-Thomson M, Pring T (1990) The use of picture/word matching tasks to assist word retrieval in aphasic patients. Aphasiology 4: 167–84.

Morris J (1997) Word deafness: a comparison of auditory and semantic treatments. Unpublished PhD thesis. University of York.

Nickels LA, Best W (1996a) Therapy for naming deficits (part I): Principles, puzzles and progress. Aphasiology 10: 21–47.

Nickels LA, Best W (1996b) Therapy for naming deficits (part II): Specifics, surprises and suggestions. Aphasiology 10: 109–36.

Scott C (1987) Cognitive neuropsychological remediation of acquired language disorders. Unpublished MPhil thesis. Birkbeck College: University of London.

CHAPTER 6

Semantic processing problems of older adults

SUSAN KEMPER AND LAUREEN O'HANLON

The semantic processing problems of older adults have been extensively investigated from a number of different theoretical orientations. The cognitive ageing perspective has tended to focus on the effects of ageing on semantic memory, examining the speed of semantic priming and the mechanisms of word retrieval. More psycholinguistic investigations have extended this focus to sentence and discourse processing studies in order to investigate how ageing affects semantic aspects of comprehension and recall. Language production studies have drawn from sociolinguistic as well as psycholinguistic paradigms to investigate how ageing affects discourse coherence and referential communication. This research has documented age invariance as well as age differences, which have implicated a variety of different mechanisms including working memory limitations, general slowing, and inhibitory breakdown. This chapter reviews production and comprehension problems of older adults and concludes with some general remarks regarding explanatory mechanisms.

Production problems

Word-finding problems are among the most frequent complaints of older adults. Pauses, circumlocutions, 'empty speech' such as pronouns lacking clear referents, and substitution errors during spontaneous speech may all reflect age-related impairments in accessing and retrieving lexical information (Cohen, 1979; Obler, 1980; Ulatowska, Cannito, Hayashi et al., 1985). It appears that older adults have difficulty accessing lexical information, especially the phonological form of words (Burke, MacKay, Worthley et al., 1991). Consequently, tip-of-the-tongue experiences, in which familiar words are temporarily irretrievable, are more common for older adults than for young adults and less often resolved by retrieval of the intended word. Word-finding problems are also apparent in controlled tasks such as requiring word retrieval given definitions (Bowles, Obler, and Albert, 1987; Bowles, Obler, and Poon, 1989; Bowles and Poon, 1981; Bowles and Poon, 1985), pictures (Albert, Heller, and Milberg, 1988; Nicholas, Obler, Albert et al., 1985), or category cues (Howard, Shaw, and Heisey, 1986; Obler and Albert, 1981). Evidence of word retrieval difficulties has also been found during picture and video description tasks (Heller and Dobbs, 1993).

Name retrieval is a particularly troubling word-finding difficulty for older adults (Burke and Laver, 1990; Cohen, 1994; Cohen and Faulkner, 1986). This selective deficit for proper names does not seem to reflect specific changes in the cognitive system (Cohen, 1994). Some evidence suggests that the interaction of low levels of cognitive activation in older people may affect face and/or voice identification (Maylor, 1990, 1993, 1997) due to cognitive slowing or working memory deficits, and the lexical distinctiveness of proper names (Burton and Bruce, 1992; Cohen, 1990). That is, because proper names have fewer semantic associations than other words and because proper names are phonologically highly similar, normative word-finding difficulties experienced by older persons are increased whenever the desired word is a proper name. Although the evidence appears consistent, one recent study (Maylor, 1997) has concluded that name retrieval is not disproportionally affected by ageing though it nonetheless remains a persistent source of concern for older adults.

Despite the current controversy, anecdotal evidence indicates that proper nouns – especially proper names – are more difficult to retrieve than common nouns (Cohen, 1990a). Research of natural and experimentally induced word retrieval failures or tip-of-the-tongue (TOT) episodes also indicates that proper names are significantly more difficult to retrieve than common nouns (Burke et al., 1991; Cohen and Faulkner, 1986). Burke et al.(1991) studied diary responses from groups of young, middle age, and older adults and found significantly more reports of TOTs for proper nouns across all age groups. Burke et al. (1991) and Cohen and Faulkner (1986) also demonstrated through experimental designs that proper nouns are more susceptible to TOTs and these differences increase with age.

Young, Hay and Ellis (1985) and Schweich, van der Linden, Bredart et al. (1992) examined diary responses from subjects and concluded that names are typically retrieved following prior activation of some level of identity-specific semantic information. Other experimental data (Hay, Young and Ellis, 1991) also indicates that prior activation of some semantic information is likely before proper nouns are retrieved.

McWeeney, Young, Hay et al. (1987) demonstrated that, even when word forms were equivalent (*Baker* versus *baker*), words presented as names (*Baker*) were more difficult to recall than words presented as occupations (*baker*). Overall, lexical access demonstrates a strong preference for general semantic information whereas proper nouns appear separate and secondary to these general semantic structures. Several models of lexical access have been proposed to explain these differences in word retrieval.

Bruce and Young (1986) developed a model of lexical access to account for the specific processes of proper name retrieval. In this model (Figure 1), a person is recognized through an encoding of visual and contextual features. This visual recognition centre leads to the activation of a person identity node (PIN). A PIN includes semantic information stored about the particular person, known as identity-specific semantic codes. Activation of the PIN leads to the final stage of activating the person's name via the name node. The person's name is not activated until the PIN has been activated and some amount of semantic information is retrieved.

By representing access to names with a single connection always subsequent to some level of semantic and subsequent PIN activation, this model attempts to account for the delayed access to names as compared to retrieval of other biographical information which does not require the PIN activation.

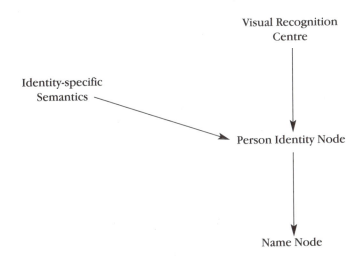

Adapted from Bruce V, Young A (1986) Understanding face recognition. British Journal of Psychology 77: 305–27.

Figure 1. A model of proper name retrieval.

The Bruce and Young (1986) model is a hierarchical serially ordered model. The name node is activated only through the activation of the PIN and there is no feedback through the system. Burton and Bruce (1993) developed an interactive version of the Bruce and Young model (Figure 2). In this model, the semantic information about the person is stored in the semantic system while the PINs are considered access nodes to the semantic system (Valentine, Brennen and Bredart, 1996). Names are no longer considered a separate node but represent an entry in the semantic system. Burton and Bruce (1993) suggest increased difficulties with proper names are due to a single link between the PIN and the name within the semantic system. Because other information represented in the semantic system has multiple connections to other related PINs, they receive spreading activation and are more quickly and easily activated compared to names.

Burke et al. (1991) proposed a model (Figures 3 and 4) of lexical access which explains the advantage of common nouns over proper nouns in terms of the node structure theory (MacKay and Burke, 1990). Like the Burton and Bruce (1993) interactive model, this model focuses on the convergence of connectivity within the semantic system. In the Burke et al.(1991) model, the level of activation of particular lexical item depends upon the number of converging connections on a particular lexical node (MacKay and Burke, 1990). Common nouns have many semantic information nodes activated which converge on the lexical node for that word (Figure 3).

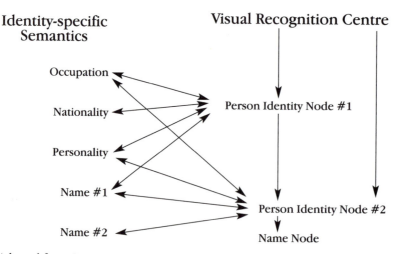

Adapted from Burton AM, Bruce V (1993) I recognise your face but I can't remember your name: a simple explanation? British Journal of Psychology 83: 45–60.

Figure 2. An interactive model of proper name retrieval.

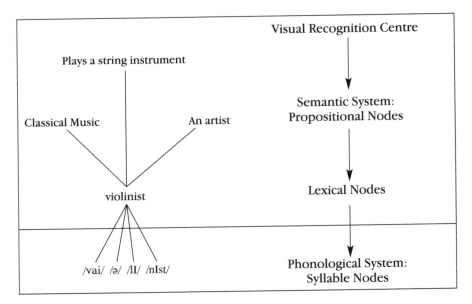

Adapted from Burke DM, Mackay DG, Worthley JS, Wade E (1991) On the tip of the tongue: what causes word finding failures in young and older adults. Journal of Memory and Language 30: 542–79.

Figure 3. A model of common noun retrieval.

The word *violinist* is activated by the convergence of priming received from the various semantic nodes connected to it (e.g. plays a string instrument, an artist). The semantic information for proper nouns (Figure 4), however, converges on a proper name node, which in turn diverges to individual lexical nodes for first and second names. Retrieving the name of a violinist and next door neighbour, Alicia Brown, will activate some of the same semantic information, but Burke et al. argue that the single link between the proper name node and the individual names will not transmit as much priming as the multiple links from semantic nodes to the common noun lemma.

Recently, Valentine, Brennan, and Bredart (1996) proposed a model of lexical access which attempts to integrate all three of these perspectives (Figure 5). To explain the differences in proper and common noun retrieval, this model establishes two pathways of lexical access for common nouns versus proper nouns. Common nouns are accessed through the activation of the semantic system and subsequent lexical nodes. Activating the semantic lexicon involves retrieval of what Levelt (1989) referred to as 'lemmas'. Lemmas are semantic representations that do not include any information regarding phonological form but they do

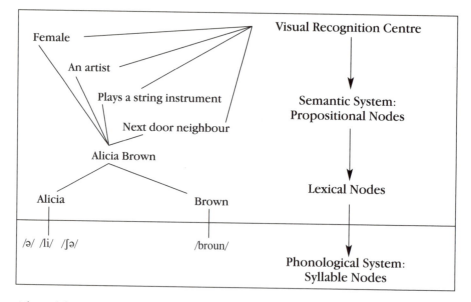

Adapted from Burke DM, Mackay DG, Worthley JS, Wade E (1991) On the tip of the tongue: what causes word finding failures in young and older adults. Journal of Memory and Language 30: 542–79.

Figure 4. A model of proper name retrieval.

contain information regarding grammatical class. For example, retrieving the lemma of 'violinist' would include retrieving the information that it is a noun capable of serving as a subject or an object of an argument structure. This initial stage of lexical access triggers the activation of the lexemes (Levelt, 1989) for the particular common noun. Lexemes are word representations that include phonological information. According to Valentine et al. (1996), proper nouns are accessed through a route separate from common noun information. Proper nouns are accessed directly from a person identity node. The PIN acts as a unit of recognition of the person and serves to activate the proper noun lemma for that person. The proper noun lemma is a non-lexical specification of the name. Proper noun lemmas are activated through a single connection from the PIN. This proper noun lemma then triggers the activation of the lexical-phono-logical forms or lexemes. Access to proper nouns does not benefit from the converging activation of the semantic system on the lemma for a common noun. For example, in Figure 5, the common noun 'violinist' is activated following a convergence of semantic associates which add together to provide enough priming to activate the lemma for 'violinist.' However, the violinist's name, 'Alicia', is activated without the benefit of semantic associates with only a single connection from the PIN to the proper noun lemma. Valentine et al. (1996) argue that this single link between the PIN and the name lemmas is the reason for decreased transmission of priming with even less priming spreading to individual first and last names.

Overall, the primary distinction between accessing proper versus common nouns in all of these models is converging activation from semantic nodes to common nouns but single or divergent connections to proper names. In all four models, lemmas for proper nouns are set apart either in a separated semantic store or by decreased interactive connections. Based on this, these models make similar predictions regarding retrieval of proper versus common nouns. These models predict that common nouns will be easier to retrieve than proper nouns and that access to proper nouns is more susceptible to decrements due to minimal linkage strength. A primary source of decrement is age and therefore these models predict that the efficiency or proper noun retrieval will likely decrease with age.

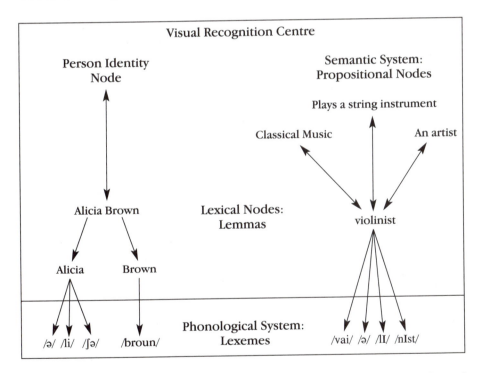

Adapted from Valentine T, Brennen T, Bredart S (1996) The Cognitive Psychology of Proper Names. London: Routledge.

Figure 5. A model of proper name and common noun retrieval.

As already noted, the evidence currently suggests that word retrieval abilities change with age. Au, Joung, Nicholas et al. (1995) found a steady decline in word retrieval skills throughout the lifespan. Burke et al.(1991) demonstrated through diary and experimental studies that older adults exhibit more TOT states than younger adults for common and proper nouns. Diary studies and questionnaires indicate that older adults experience more TOTs for peoples' names than any other word category (Burke et al., 1991; Cohen and Faulkner, 1984). These changes in word retrieval abilities do not, however, coincide with evidence of loss in semantic memory. There is consistent evidence throughout the ageing literature that vocabulary scores are higher for older adults than younger and semantic priming effects demonstrate no significant changes in the structure of the semantic lexicon (Light, 1991; Light and Burke, 1988). Word retrieval deficits do not appear to be related to impaired storage of information but rather to ineffective access. Several theories of word retrieval deficits have been proposed but few have provided significant clarity to understanding age differences.

Cohen and Faulkner (1986) proposed that names are more difficult to retrieve because they involve retrieval of one specific label, whereas a common noun can often be represented with synonyms. The specificity of name retrieval may require more time to access than retrieving any number of synonyms for a particular common noun. Bredart (1993) examined the effects of retrieving names of individuals associated with two well-known names (e.g. Harrison Ford associated with Indiana Jones) versus those with one name (Julia Roberts). This study demonstrated fewer word retrieval blocks when there were two names available for access. It seems plausible that older adults exhibit increased word retrieval deficits, particularly for proper names, due to the difficulty in accessing one particular item in the lexicon. Yet this position does not explain why all words are subject to increased retrieval deficits with age. In fact, since older adults demonstrate increased vocabulary compared to younger adults (Light, 1991) then they should have many more synonymous choices and overall word retrieval should improve with age.

Cohen (1990b) proposed that proper nouns are difficult to retrieve because they are not meaningful. This idea is directly related to the model representations of Valentine et al. (1996) and Burke et al. (1991) that separate proper nouns from other semantic or biographical information. Cohen (1990b) demonstrated that meaningless non-words about an individual were just as difficult to recall as learning their names, for example, 'This is Mr. Collins. He has a "wesp".' The evidence indicated that the advantage of common nouns was related to their semantic representations, and proper nouns or non-words are arbitrarily connected to people with no significant semantic support for their connection. This position may readily explain age differences in word retrieval based on significant evidence that older adults benefit from semantic context and relatedness (Light, 1991, Light and Burke, 1988).

Another proposal explains that the word retrieval problem is due to the size of the plausible phonology for a particular lemma. Brennan (1993) proposed that proper nouns are more difficult to retrieve because names have a larger number of possible phonological representations than common nouns. This set size of plausible phonologies acts in a top-down processing manner. When a word is being accessed for production, higher-level knowledge may indicate that it is a common or highly familiar word. This knowledge will constrain the size of plausible phonologies that will be activated for that word. On the other hand, when a proper noun is accessed, the top-down constraints do not restrict the SSPP because names can be represented by a large number of possible phonological strings. This proposal targets processes of phonological access as the main cause of word retrieval deficits for proper nouns. This explanation appears somewhat more consistent with the fact that older adults show increased word retrieval deficits alongside increased vocabulary. It is plausible that as vocabularies expand through exposure to more and more names over the years, older adults develop larger SSPP which impairs access across all words, especially proper nouns.

There is one theoretical proposal that provides an integrative perspective across all of these positions. Burke et al. (1991) proposed that increased word retrieval deficits in older adults are caused by reduced transmission of priming based on the node structure theory (MacKay and Burke, 1990). They argue that language production, in contrast to language comprehension, is a process of convergent to divergent activation. Words are produced through a converging of semantic activation upon a lexical node followed by a divergent activation of the phonological nodes representing the form of the word. This divergent activation is an example of a single source factor. A single source factor is 'when a node critical to a task receives priming from only a single source or connection within the network' (MacKay and Burke, 1990: p 251). Phonological nodes for a particular lemma will receive priming from a single connection to the activated lemma (see Figure 5); there is no advantage of convergence or summation of priming to facilitate access and therefore these connections are susceptible to decreased activation or retrieval failures. Proper nouns exhibit a higher level of single source activation between the person identity node and the lemma for proper nouns making them even more vulnerable to impaired activation. Under the node structure theory, the transmission deficit hypothesis proposes that 'age weakens the linkage strength of connections between nodes in the network so that rate and asymptotic amount of priming transmitted across any given connection declines with age' (MacKay and Burke, 1990: p 221). Because the lexical access system for language production includes single source connections between semantic and phonological nodes, word retrieval is particularly vulnerable to age-related transmission deficits. Because proper nouns have multiple levels of single source connections, they are even more vulnerable to the effects of ageing on the transmission of priming.

The transmission deficit hypothesis can incorporate many of these theoretical proposals regarding proper noun difficulties. If names are more difficult to retrieve because they involve retrieval of one specific label (Cohen and Faulkner, 1986), this indicates a single vulnerable connection from the conceptual node to the specific label (lemma) without benefit from summation of priming from other related forms. If names are more difficult because they lack meaning (Cohen, 1990b), this also indicates a single connection from some type of conceptual identification node (or PIN) to the proper noun lemma without benefit of converging priming from a rich semantic network. Finally, if names are more difficult to retrieve because of the size of the plausible phonology (Brennan, 1992), this points to the issue of divergent spread of priming through a large phonological store.

The transmission deficit hypothesis is also supported by phonological priming research. Phonological priming effects on word retrieval have been explored through priming experiments where participants are given phonological or semantic cues to facilitate word retrieval (Brennan et al., 1990; Meyer and Bock, 1992). These experiments indicate that younger adults may benefit more from phonological than semantic cues. This is consistent with the view that the divergent activation of phonological information is the weak link in word retrieval and when this is facilitated, word retrieval improves. Age differences in phonological effects of word retrieval have not been examined specifically.

Word retrieval problems are but one indication of how ageing affects older adults' semantic processing. Semantic processing problems may also affect other aspects of older adults' discourse, including their ability to perform referential communication tasks and the occurrence of off-target verbosity. There is some evidence that discourse skills improve with age. Older adults create elaborate narrative structures that include hierarchically detailed episodes. These narratives often include beginnings which describe initiating events and motivating states, developments which detail the protagonist's goals and actions, and endings which summarize the outcomes of the protagonist's efforts. Older adults also tend to attach evaluative codas to assess the contemporary significance of these stories

(Kemper and Anagnopoulos, 1989; Kemper, Rash, Kynette et al., 1990; Pratt, Boyes, Robins et al., 1989; Pratt and Robins, 1991; but see also Juncos-Rabadan, 1996, and Juncos-Rabadan and Iglesias, 1994). Narrative stories told by older adults are evaluated more positively, preferred by listeners, and are more memorable than those told by young adults (James, Burke, Austin et al., 1998; Kemper and Anagnopoulos, 1989; Kemper et al., 1990; Pratt et al., 1989; Pratt and Robins, 1991).

In contrast, older adults often have difficulty with referential communication tasks. In one such referential communication task, Hupet, Chantraine and Nef (1993) tracked how dyads of young and older adults formulated mutually acceptable labels for abstract drawings. The older adults benefited less from repetition of the task than the young adults; whereas the young adults added new information to previously used descriptions, the older adults tended to supply totally new labels. The older adults' problems with this task may have resulted from forgetting of the old labels from trial to trial or from their inability to inhibit irrelevant thoughts or associations, including the new descriptions.

In a series of studies, Kemper and her colleagues (Kemper, Othick, Gerhing et al., 1996; Kemper, Othick, Warren et al., 1998; Kemper, Vandeputte, Rice et al., 1995) have compared young–young, old–old, and young–old dyads on a referential communication task involving giving map directions. Whereas young adults spontaneously adopt a simplified speech style when addressing older adults versus age-equivalent peers, older adults do not appear to code-switch. This may be due to a number of factors:

1. Older adults may not be sensitive to the same situational cues that elicit code-switching from the young adults.
2. Older adults may not be able to vary their grammatical complexity or semantic content while simultaneously executing the complex task.
3. Older speakers may have 'optimized' their speech to peers as a result of extensive practice at communicating with other older adults and adults experiencing communicative problems; hence, shifting to a non-optimal speech style when addressing younger adults would not be an appropriate strategy.
4. Older adults may be unwilling to shift to a simplified speech style when they are addressing peers since this form of speech may resemble patronizing talk (Ryan, Hummert, and Boich, 1995) or secondary baby talk (Caporael, 1981).
5. Semantic processing problems, especially problems with word retrieval, may interfere with and limit older adults' ability to employ code-switching.

The last hypothesis is supported by other indications that older adults' discourse is affected by semantic processing problems. For example, conversations with older adults are often marked by 'painful self-disclosures' of bereavement, ill-health, immobility, and assorted personal and family problems (Coupland, Coupland, and Giles, 1991). From an interpersonal point of view, painful self-disclosures may serve several different goals for communicators (Coupland, Coupland, and Grainger, 1991; Shaner, 1996), for example, maintaining 'face' by contrasting personal strengths and competencies with past problems and limitations, and coping with personal losses and difficulties. Yet painful self-disclosures also maintain and reinforce negative age stereotypes about the elderly as weak and disabled (Shaner, 1996). Consequently, such self-disclosures can suppress conversational interactions and limit the quality of intergenerational communication (Nussbaum, Hummert, Williams et al., 1996). From a processing point of view, painful self-disclosures may arise from the persistent intrusion of thoughts due to chronic activation within the semantic memory network.

A final discourse style often presumed to accompany ageing is verbosity, or repetitious, prolonged, off-target speech. Verbosity may arise from a breakdown of inhibitory processes within the semantic memory network. However, recent research (Arbuckle and Gold, 1993; Arbuckle, Gold, and Andres, 1986; Gold, Andres, Arbuckle et al., 1988; Gold and Arbuckle, 1992, 1995; Gold, Arbuckle, and Andres, 1994) has suggested that verbosity is not a general characteristic of older adults but is an extreme form of talkativeness that results from intellectual decline associated with frontal lobe impairments (see Arbuckle and Gold, 1993, for a review of these issues). Frontal lobe impairments disrupt inhibitory processes and lead to preseverative behaviours on other tasks. Verbosity can be characterized as involving a loss of the ability to inhibit competing responses; hence, an age-related loss of frontal lobe function may lead to increased verbosity among older adults. Verbosity, like talk of the past, painful self-disclosures and age disclosures, may disrupt social interactions and lead to a loss of interpersonal contact and social support. Unlike the other semantic processing problems of older adults, however, verbosity appears to reflect changes in semantic processes that lie at the juncture between normal and pathological ageing.

Comprehension problems

The encoding of perceptual characteristics of words, such as phonetic and graphemic properties, does not appear to decline with age (Naveh-Benjamin and Craik, 1995). However, older adults have processing difficulties when these features depart from normal. Ferraro and Kellas (1992) and Ferraro (1994) examined how the perceptual characteristics of letter strings, when presented at 0, 30, 60 or more degrees from upright, influenced older adults' reaction times in a semantically primed lexical decision task. Both studies showed that older participants' responses were considerably slowed for letter strings that were beyond the 30 degree orientation mark compared with younger participants who processed the 30 and 60 degree strings as well as those presented at the 0 degree mark. Another study, using a word-stem completion task, found that typeface variations (i.e. whether or not the typeface of the words on the study list matched the typeface of the to-be-completed stem) did not differentially influence older adults' responses in a sentence or letter judgement task (Gibson, Brooks, Friedman et al., 1993). Further, Madden (1992) examined younger and older adults' reaction times to singly-primed targets in a lexical decision task and demonstrated a larger age-related effect of slowing for visually degraded targets relative to non-degraded targets. Sommers (1996) has extended this argument by showing that older adults have greater difficulty identifying lexically difficult words. Lexical difficulty was defined by two properties of words: neighbourhood density, or the number of phonetically similar words, and neighbourhood frequency, the average occurrence frequency of similar words. Perceptually and lexically difficult words may be difficult for older adults to identify because competing candidate items cannot be eliminated as readily or as rapidly due to a breakdown of inhibitory processes (Hasher and Zacks, 1988) or general slowing of cognitive processes (Salthouse, 1996) although support for either the inhibitory breakdown or general slowing theory is inclusive (Light, 1991).

Although adults' word-finding difficulties tend to increase with age, the overall representation of lexical knowledge does not appear to decline with age. The stability of lexical knowledge has been established in the context of lexical ambiguity (Kellas, Paul, and Vu, 1995), word frequency (Allen, Madden, Weber et al., 1993), and semantic relatedness (Stern, Prather, Swinney et al., 1991). Further, studies of semantic priming, in which the identification of a target (e.g., doctor) is facilitated by the prior presentation of a semantically-related prime (e.g., nurse), have shown relatively few age differences (e.g. Balota and Duchek, 1988; but see Laver and Burke, 1993). Tests of individual word identification and word stem or fragment completion have generally shown that older adults' access to lexical information, while sometimes slower, is comparable to that of younger adults (Light and Singh, 1987; Burke, White, and Diaz, 1987; Madden, 1986; Madden, Pierce, and Allen, 1993; but see Chiarello and Hoyer, 1988; Hultsch, Masson, and Small, 1991). This type of effect suggests that the semantic association of lexical items remains fairly stable in older adulthood.

Several researchers have challenged the view that lexical knowledge remains well preserved in ageing. Myerson, Ferraro, Hale et al. (1992) analysed data from studies on semantic priming, word naming, and pronunciation and showed that there is a proportional relationship between older and younger adults' priming effects of approximately 1.5. This finding is in line with a meta-analysis by Laver and Burke (1993) which found that priming effects are larger for older adults. These studies suggest that while the structure of lexical information may be intact, access to the information declines proportionally with age.

Semantic processing problems may also be at the root of older adults' text processing problems. Wingfield and colleagues have focused on empirical investigations of how the semantic (or propositional), syntactic, and prosodic structures of speech influence adults' auditory comprehension of discourse. Wingfield and Stine (1986), for example, found that older adults, like young, segmented auditory-based prose at syntactic boundaries and that recall performance did not decline as the rate of presentation increased. Stine, Wingfield, and Poon (1986) tested whether increased propositional density of text and increased presentation rates disrupted older adults' recall of auditorily presented text. Stine et al. found that older adults were not differentially influenced by the high propositionally dense text, though their recall performance was poorest for speeded text presentation. In a reanalysis of the Stine et al. (1986) data, Stine and Wingfield (1988) compared the qualitative nature of younger and older adults' recall of the propositionally dense sentences. Stine and Wingfield found that, as propositional density increased, older adults were less likely to recall the same main-story ideas as younger adults. Thompson (1995) has shown that older adults benefit from seeing visual cues for the articulation of speech when tested with meaningful or anomalous sentences. In contrast, when Stine, Wingfield, and Myers (1990) examined younger and older adults' recall of information from a television newscast, visual presentation did not improve older adults' recall. Lip-reading may benefit older adults, but they may be unable to sustain this skill for extended periods or when processing complex discourse.

Older adults' processing of written text may also be limited by semantic processing problems. The comprehension of short phrases does not appear to decline with age but as the text and text processing demands increase, age differences begin to appear. Hess, Flannagan, and Tate (1993) examined adults' organization and recall of taxonomically organized phrases (e.g. vehicles category: 'get on bus' and 'ride on train') versus schematically organized phrases (e.g. going to work activities: 'ride on train' and 'go in office'). Older adults' recall of phrases was best for schematically organized phrases relative to taxonomically organized phrases; however, older adults did not differentially benefit from the organization relative to younger adults, suggesting that older adults are able to integrate such short phrases. Hess (1995) extended this approach to pairs of sentences such as 'Cathy felt very dizzy and fainted at her work. She was carried unconscious to the hospital.' Older adults were less likely to spontaneously generate appropriate causal connections between such sentence pairs; as a result, they were less likely to recall the second sentence of the pair when prompted with the first. LaVoie and Malmstrom (1998) also suggested that older adults have difficulty spontaneously infer-ring thematically consistent causal connections and, as a consequence, are less likely to falsely recognize actions that are consistent with a story.

The studies of older adults' text and prose processing have largely shown that text-level characteristics, such as semantic or propositional content and syntactic structure greatly influence older adults' text compre-hension (see Light and Burke, 1988, for comprehensive reviews). For example, Zelinski, Light, and Gilewski (1984) have found that older and younger adults recalled qualitatively similar features of the expository text – though older adults recalled less information than younger adults. Though overall recall of propositionally dense text may be unimpaired, older adults tend to recall fewer main ideas relative to younger adults (Stine and Wingfield, 1988) and to allocate less reading time to propositionally dense sentences (Stine and Hindman, 1994). Researchers have also documented deficits in older adults' ability to identify pronominal referents as text processing loads increase (Light and Capps, 1986; Morrow, Altieri and Leirer, 1992; Morrow, Leirer and Altieri, 1992; but see also Light, Capps, Singh et al., 1994) and generate inferences from text (Cohen, 1979; Zacks, Hasher, Doren et al., 1987; but see Zelinski, 1988). Connelly, Hasher and Zacks (1991) and Dywan and Murphy (1996) suggest that older adults' text processing difficulties may be due to reduced inhibitory control: while reading short paragraphs, older adults are less able to ignore distractors, such as words printed in a different type font.

Recent research on text comprehension in ageing has focused on the text- and reader-level variables that influence processing as it takes place or online. Hartley, Stojack, Mushaney et al. (1994) compared younger and older adults' recall of prose which was presented in experimenter- and self-paced presentation rates. They found that older adults recalled less than younger adults as the time available for processing increased. At the text level, Stine (1990) found that younger and older adults allocated word-by-word reading times similarly for word-level and more global phrase-level features of the text. Younger adults allocated additional reading time to the ends of phrases, clauses, and sentences whereas older adults' reading times were longer at clause boundaries. A related study by Stine, Cheung, and Henderson (1995) extended this earlier research by showing that specific word-, phrase-, sentence-, and discourse-level features of text influenced older adults' word-by-word reading times and explicit recall of narrative texts such that, overall, older adults tended to allocate less reading time to processing new concepts. Stine, Loveless, and Soederberg (1996) demonstrated that younger and older adults' on–line reading times were qualitatively similar in that both age groups allocated more reading time to text sectors with complex syntax, new concepts, and longer words. In contrast, older adults allocated less reading time, relative to young, for new concepts. A recent study by Soederberg Miller and Stine-Morrow (1998) compared reading time allocation strategies for older adults who achieve high levels of recall and those who exhibit recall deficits. When challenged by vague, ill-defined texts, older readers may be able to maintain high levels of recall by allocating additional processing time to new concepts and complex syntactic constructions, especially when they are able to draw upon background knowledge triggered by an informative title. Morrow, Stine-Morrow, Leirer et al. (1997) also found that older adults differentially slow down when reading narratives in order to achieve a high level of recall. Stine-Morrow and her colleagues suggest that older adults may compensate for working memory declines by adopting processing strategies that parse a text into smaller units and by relying on background knowledge in order to integrate these units. When such background information is available, older readers who adopt such processing strategies may have few difficulties processing narrative prose (Radvansky and Curiel, 1998).

Older adults' discourse processing problems may affect real-world behaviours, such as understanding medication instructions (Morrow, Hier, Menard et al., 1998) and making decisions about medical treatment for breast cancer. Meyer, Russo, and Talbot (1996) studied how younger and older women process textual information about breast cancer treatments. Older women make decisions about treatment more rapidly than younger women: older women spend less time seeking out, reading, and analysing medical information. Meyer et al. (1996) suggest that older women may be motivated to make a decision quickly in order to reduce cognitive demands during stressful periods.

Conclusions

In sum, although age deficits in semantic processing, especially word retrieval, are well documented, age invariance has also been observed for many aspects of language production and comprehension. Two theoretical perspectives have emerged in recent years regarding the occurrence or non-occurrence of age deficits on production and comprehension. On one hand, some have attributed age deficits in language processing to an age-related decline in the capacity of working memory; hence, age deficits are to be expected whenever processing task demands exceed older adults' working memory. Processing strategies that reduce task demands, such as segmenting texts into smaller processing units (Stine, Loveless, and Soederberg, 1996), may enable older readers to achieve high levels of text recall. The processing of complex syntactic constructions has traditionally been assumed to impose severe demands on working memory for the simultaneous storage and manipulation of syntactic constituents (Chomsky, 1957; Gibson and Thomas, 1996; King and Just, 1991); hence, Kemper (1992) and Just and Carpenter (1992) suggested that age deficits in syntactic processing, arising from working memory limitations, may contribute to more general text processing problems of older adults. Waters and Caplan (1996a, 1996b, 1996c) have challenged this view, based in part on recent studies comparing adults differing in working memory capacity, such as that by Kemtes and Kemper (1997). This study, in conjunction with those of Stine-Morrow and her colleagues, suggests that immediate syntactic processing appears to be age-invariant although post-interpretive processes, required for text integration and discourse comprehension, may be vulnerable to age-related effects of working memory deficits.

A breakdown of inhibitory processes has also been suggested as a general mechanism underlying age deficits in production and comprehension by Hasher and Zacks (1988). This view is supported by findings such as those by Connelly, Hasher, and Zacks (1991) and Dywan and Murphy (1996) showing that older adults are less able to ignore irrelevant, distracting information while reading; there are also reports of an age-related increase in off-task verbosity (e.g. Arbuckle and Gold, 1993). Kwong See and Ryan (1995) examined individual differences in text processing attributable to working memory capacity (Stine, 1990), efficiency of inhibitory processes (Gernsbacher, 1990), and processing speed (Cohen, 1979), estimated by backward digit span, colour naming speed, and Stroop interference respectively. Their analysis suggested that working memory capacity is correlated with processing speed and inhibitory efficiency and that older adults' language processing difficulties can be attributed, at least in part, to the slower processing and less efficient inhibition. However, this view has been challenged by Burke (1997; but see Zacks and Hasher, 1997, for a reply). Burke argues that a variety of different explanations are required to account for these phenomena: other memory deficits may contribute to older adults' poor performance on the post-comprehension tests used by Connelly et al. and Dywan and Murphy, whereas verbosity may reflect a distinct speech style adopted in some social contexts by both young and older adults.

MacKay and Burke (1990) have recently proposed an integrative theory which identifies linguistic units like other cognitive units as organized into nodes. These nodes are linked to other nodes in a system of priming and activation. A particular node will vary in its readiness for activation by the degree of priming received or spread from other nodes throughout the linkage system. Although priming spreads and summates on individual nodes, activation is an all-or-none phenomenon which does not spread. Linkages between nodes are strengthened by frequency of activation so that a particular set of nodes are more likely to reach summation of priming and therefore become activated if they or their linked nodes have recently been activated. MacKay and Burke (1990) conclude that ageing leads to reduced spread of priming due to weak linkages throughout the whole cognitive system and linguistically this is most significant in reduced efficiency of language production.

According to Abrams and MacKay (1998), language production systems may be more vulnerable to ageing because production relies on a divergence of activation across a large set of possible nodes whereas comprehension requires only the convergence of information on to a smaller set of potential nodes. This divergence of activation in production means that language processing moves from a small set of concepts in the mind to a large set of possible combinations of linguistic units. Convergence of activation in comprehension, however, means that processing moves from a large set of linguistic inputs to a smaller set of potential concepts related to that input.

This position may have the potential of integrating many of the current findings in language and ageing research. The node structure theory has been proposed to explain age-related differences in word retrieval, new versus old learning, and effects of ambiguity (MacKay and Burke, 1990). The basis of hypothesized age-related differences is that any behaviour that utilizes single-source factors is vulnerable to reduced efficiency of priming with age. Single-source factors are divergent single connections to essential information which when lost or weakened will lead to a failure in the behaviour. Word retrieval failures are considered a strong example of a single-source factor with divergent spreading of priming occurring during phonological access. Proper name retrieval is an even stronger example since names are accessed through a single connection between the PIN and the proper name lemma.

Acknowledgements

Preparation of this chapter was supported by grant RO1 AG0092 from the National Institute on Aging to Susan Kemper and by the Research Training Program in Communication and Aging, grant RO1 AG000226. O'Hanlon is now with the Department of Speech-Language-Hearing, University of California-Davis.

References

Abrams L, MacKay DG (1998) Age-linked asymmetries in the detection and retrieval of orthographic information. Poster presented at the Cognitive Aging Conference, April 1998: Atlanta, GA.

Albert MS, Heller HS, Milberg W (1988) Changes in naming ability with age. Psychology and Aging 3: 173–78.

Allen PA, Madden DJ, Weber TA, Groth KE (1993) Influence of age and processing stage on visual word recognition. Psychology and Aging 8: 274–82.

Arbuckle TY, Gold DP (1993) Aging inhibition and verbosity. Journal of Gerontology: Psychological Sciences 48: 225–32.

Arbuckle TY Gold DP, Andres D (1986) Cognitive functioning of older people in relation to social and personality variables. Psychology and Aging 1: 55–62.

Au R, Joung P, Nicholas M, Obler LK (1995) Naming ability across the adult life span. Aging and Cognition 2: 300–11.

Balota DA, Duchek JM (1988) Age-related differences in lexical access spreading activation and simple pronunciation time. Psychology and Aging 3: 84–93.

Bowles NL, Obler LK, Albert ML (1987) Naming errors in healthy aging and dementia of the Alzheimer type. Cortex 23: 519–24.

Bowles NL, Obler LK, Poon LW (1989) Aging and word retrieval: naturalistic clinical and laboratory data. In Poon LW, Rubin DC, Wilson BA, (Eds) Everyday Cognition in Adulthood and Late Life. New York: Cambridge University Press.

Bowles NL, Poon LW (1981) The effect of age on speed of lexical access. Experimental Aging Research 7: 417–25.

Bowles NL, Poon LW (1985) Aging and the retrieval of words in semantic memory. Journal of Gerontology 40: 71–77.

Bredart S (1993) Retrieval failures in face naming. Memory 1: 351–66.

Brennan T (1992) The difficulty with recalling people's names: the plausible phonology hypothesis. Memory 1: 409–31.

Brennan T, Baguley T, Bright J, Bruce V (1990) Resolving semantically induced tip-of-the-tongue states for proper nouns. Memory and Cognition 18: 339–47.

Bruce V, Young A (1986) Understanding face recognition. British Journal of Psychology 77: 305–27.

Burke D (1997) Language, aging and inhibitory deficits: evaluation of a theory. Journal of Gerontology: Psychological Sciences 52B: 254–64.

Burke DM, Laver GD (1990) Aging and word retrieval: selective age deficits in language. In Lovelace EA, (Ed) Aging and Cognition: Mental Processes, Self-awareness and Interventions. New York: Elsevier-North Holland.

Burke DM, MacKay DG, Worthley JS, Wade E (1991) On the tip of the tongue: what causes word finding failures in young and older adults. Journal of Memory and Language 30: 542–79.

Burke DM, White H, Diaz DL (1987) Semantic priming in young and older adults: evidence for age constancy in automatic and attentional processes. Journal of Experimental Psychology: Human Perception and Performance 13: 78–88.

Burton AM, Bruce V (1992) I recognize your face but I can't remember your name: a simple explanation? British Journal of Psychology 83: 45–60.

Burton A M, Bruce V (1993) Naming faces and naming names: exploring an interactive activation model of name retrieval. Memory 1: 457–80.

Caporael L (1981) The paralanguage of caregiving: baby talk to the institutionalized aged. Journal of Personality and Social Psychology 40: 876–84.

Chiarello C, Hoyer WJ (1988) Adult age differences in implicit and explicit memory: time course and encoding effects: Psychology and Aging 3: 358–66.

Chomsky N (1957) Syntactic structures. The Hague: Mouton.

Cohen G (1979) Language comprehension in old age. Cognitive Psychology 11: 412–29.

Cohen G (1990a) Recognition and retrieval of proper names: age differences in the fan effect. European Journal of Cognitive Psychology 2: 193–204.

Cohen G (1990b) Why is it difficult to put names to faces? British Journal of Psychology 81: 287–97.

Cohen G (1994) Age-related problems in the use of proper names in communication. In Hummert ML, Wiemann JM, Nussbaum JF, (Eds) Interpersonal Communication in Older Adulthood: Interdisciplinary Theory and Research. Newbury Park: Sage.

Cohen G, Faulkner D (1984) Memory in old age: good in parts. New Scientist 11: 49–51.

Cohen G, Faulkner D (1986) Memory for proper names: age differences in retrieval. British Journal of Developmental Psychology 4: 187–97.

Connelly SL, Hasher L, Zacks RT (1991) Age and reading: the impact of distraction. Psychology and Aging 6: 533–41.

Coupland J, Coupland N, Giles H (1991) My life in your hands: processes of intergenerational self-disclosure. In Coupland N, Coupland J, Giles H, (Eds) Language, Society and the Elderly. Oxford: Basil Blackwell.

Coupland J, Coupland N, Grainger K (1991) Intergenerational discourse: contextual versions of ageing and elderliness. Ageing and Society II: 189–208.

Dywan J, Murphy WE (1996) Aging and inhibitory control in text comprehension. Psychology and Aging 11: 199–206.

Ferraro FR (1994) Word-unit analysis during visual word recognition in young and elderly adults. Developmental Neuropsychology 10: 13–17.

Ferraro FR, Kellas G (1992) Age-related changes in the effects of target orientation on word recognition. Journals of Gerontology 47: 279–80.

Gernsbacher MA (1990) Language comprehension as structure building. Hillsdale, NJ: Erlbaum.

Gibson E, Thomas J (1996) The processing complexity of English center-embedded and self-embedded structures. In Schultze C, (Ed) Proceedings of the NELS 26 Workshop on Language Processing. Cambridge, MA: MIT Working Papers in Linguistics.

Gibson JM, Brooks JO, Friedman L, Yesavage JA (1993) Typography manipulations can affect priming of word stem completion in older and younger adults. Psychology and Aging 8: 481–89.

Gold D, Andres D, Arbuckle T, Schwartzman A (1988) Measurement and correlates of verbosity in elderly people. Journal of Gerontology: Psychological Sciences 43: 27–33.

Gold DP, Arbuckle TY (1992) Interactions between personality and cognition and their implications for theories of aging. In Lovelace EA, (Ed) Aging and Cognition: Mental Processes, Self-awareness and Interventions. Amsterdam: North Holland.

Gold DP, Arbuckle TY (1995) A longitudinal study of off-target verbosity. Journal of Gerontology: Psychological Sciences 50B: 307–25.

Gold DP, Arbuckle TY, Andres D (1994) Verbosity in older adults. In Hummert ML, Wiemann JM, Nussbaum JF, (Eds) Interpersonal Communication in Older Adulthood: Interdisciplinary Theory and Research. Thousand Oaks, CA: Sage.

Hartley JT, Stojack CC, Mushaney TJ, Kiku-Annon TA, Lee DW (1994) Reading speed and prose memory in older and younger adults. Psychology and Aging 9: 216–23.

Hasher L, Zacks RT (1988) Working memory, comprehension, and aging: a review and a new view. In Bower GH (Ed) The Psychology of Learning and Motivation. New York: Academic Press.

Heller RB, Dobbs AR (1993) Age differences in word finding in discourse and nondiscourse situations. Psychology and Aging 8: 443–50.

Hess TM, Flannagan DA, Tate CS (1993) Aging and memory for schematically vs taxonomically organized materials. Journal of Gerontology: Psychological Sciences 48: 37–44.

Hess T (1995) Aging and the impact of causal connections on text comprehension and memory. Aging and Cognition 2: 216–30.

Hultsch DF, Masson ME, Small BJ (1991) Adult age differences in direct and indirect tests of memory. Journals of Gerontology 46: 22–30.

Howard DV, Shaw RJ, Heisey JG (1986) Aging and the time course of semantic activation. Journal of Gerontology 41: 195–203.

Hupet M, Chantraine Y, Nef F (1993) References in conversation between young and old normal adults. Psychology and Aging 8: 339–46.

James LE, Burke DM, Austin A, Hulme E (1998) Production and perception of 'verbosity' in younger and older adults. Psychology and Aging 13: 355–68.

Juncos-Rabadan O (1996) Narrative speech in the elderly: effects of age and education on telling stories. International Journal of Behavioral Development 19: 669–85.

Juncos-Rabadan O, Iglesias FJ (1994) Decline in the elderly's language: evidence from cross-linguistic data. Journal of Neurolinguistics 8: 183–90.

Just MA, Carpenter PA (1992) A capacity theory of comprehension: individual differences in working memory. Psychological Review 99: 122–49.

Kellas G, Paul ST, Vu H (1995) Aging and language performance: from isolated words to multiple sentence contexts. In Allen P, Bashore BV, (Eds) Age Differences in Word and Language Processing. Amsterdam: Elsevier Science Publishers.

Kemper S (1992) Language and aging. In Craik FIM, Salthouse TA, (Eds) Handbook of Aging and Cognition. Hillsdale, NJ: Lawrence Erlbaum.

Kemper S, Anagnopoulos C (1989) Language and aging. In Kaplan RB, (Ed) Annual Review of Applied Linguistics, Vol X. Los Angeles: American Language Institute. pp 37–50

Kemper S, Kynette D, Rash S, Sprott R, O'Brien K (1989) Life-span changes to adults' language: effects of memory and genre. Applied Psycholinguistics 10: 49–66.

Kemper S, Othick M, Gerhing H, Gubarchuk J, Billington C (1998) Practicing speech accommodations to older adults. Applied Psycholinguistics 19: 175–92.

Kemper S, Othick M, Warren J, Gubarchuk J, Gerhing H (1996) Facilitating older adults' performance on a referential communication task through speech accommodations. Aging, Neuropsychology, and Cognition 3: 37–55.

Kemper S, Rash SR, Kynette D, Norman S (1990) Telling stories: the structure of adults' narratives. European Journal of Cognitive Psychology 2: 205–28.

Kemper S, Vandeputte D, Rice K, Cheung H, Gubarchuk J (1995) Speech adjustments to aging during a referential communication task. Journal of Language and Social Psychology 14: 40–59.

Kemtes KA, Kemper S (1997) Younger and older adults' online processing of syntactically ambiguous sentences. Psychology and Aging 12: 362–71.

King J, Just MA (1991) Individual differences in syntactic processing: the role of working memory. Journal of Memory and Language 30: 580–602.

Kwong See ST, Ryan EB (1995) Cognitive mediation of adult age differences in language performance. Psychology and Aging 10: 458–68.

Laver GD, Burke DM (1993) Why do semantic priming effects increase in old age? A meta–analysis. Psychology and Aging 8: 34–43.

LaVoie DJ, Malmstrom T (1998) False recognition effects in young and older adults' memory for text passages. Journal of Gerontology: Psychological Sciences 53B: 255–62.

Levelt WJM (1989) Speaking: From Intention to Articulation. Cambridge, MA: MIT Press.

Light L (1991) Memory and aging: four hypotheses in search of data. In Rosenzweig MR, Porter LW, (Eds) Annual Review of Psychology. Palo Alto, CA: Annual Reviews.

Light LL, Burke DM (1988) Language, Memory, and Aging. New York: Cambridge University Press.

Light L, Capps JL (1986) Comprehension of pronouns in younger and older adults. Developmental Psychology 22: 580–85.

Light LL, Capps JL, Singh A, Albertson Owens SA (1994) Comprehension and use of anaphoric devices in younger and older adults. Discourse Processes 18: 77–103.

Light LL, Singh A (1987) Implicit and explicit memory in young and older adults. Journal of Experimental Psychology: Learning, Memory, and Cognition 13: 531–41.

MacKay DG, Abrams L (1996) Language memory and aging: distributed deficits and the structure of new-versus-old connections. In Birren JE, Schaie KW, (Eds) Handbook of the Psychology of Aging. San Diego: Academic Press.

MacKay DG, Burke DM (1990) Cognition and aging: a theory of new learning and the use of old connections. In Hess TM, (Ed) Aging and Cognition: Knowledge Organization and Utilization. Amsterdam: North-Holland: Elsevier Science Publishers.

Madden DJ (1986) Adult age differences in visual word recognition, semantic encoding and episodic retention. Experimental Aging Research 1: 71–78.

Madden DJ (1992) Four to ten milliseconds per year: age related slowing of visual word identification. Journal of Gerontology 47: 59–68.

Madden DJ, Pierce TW, Allen PA (1993) Age related slowing and the time course of semantic priming in visual word identification. Psychology and Aging 8: 490–507.

Maylor E (1990) Recognizing and naming faces: aging, memory retrieval, and tip of the tongue state. Journal of Gerontology 45: 215–26.

Maylor E (1993) Age blocking and tip of the tongue state. British Journal of Psychology 81: 123–34.

Maylor E (1997) Proper name retrieval in old age: converging evidence against disproportionate impairment. Aging, Neuropsychology, and Cognition 4: 211–26.

McWeeney KH, Young AW, Hay DC, Ellis AW (1987) Putting names to faces. British Journal of Psychology 78: 143–49.

Meyer AS, Bock K (1992) The tip-of-the-tongue phenomenon: blocking or partial activation? Memory and Cognition 20: 715–26.

Meyer BJF, Russo C, Talbort A (1995) Discourse comprehension and problem-solving: decisions about the treatment of breast cancer by women across the life span. Psychology and Aging 10: 84–103.

Morrow DG, Altieri P, Leirer V (1992) Aging, narrative organization, presentation mode, and referent choice strategies. Experimental Aging Research 18: 75–84.

Morrow DG, Leirer V, Altieri P (1992) Aging, expertise, and narrative processing Psychology and Aging 7: 376–88.

Morrow DG, Hier CM, Menard WE, Leirer VO (1998) Icons improve older and younger adults' comprehension of medication information. Journal of Gerontology: Psychological Sciences 53B: 240–54.

Morrow DG, Stine-Morrow EAL, Leirer VO, Andrassy JM, Kahn J (1997) The role of reader age and focus of attention in creating situation models from narratives. Journal of Gerontology: Psychological Sciences 52B: 73–80.

Myerson J, Ferraro FR, Hale S, Lima SD (1992) General slowing in semantic priming and word recognition. Psychology and Aging 7: 257–70.

Naveh-Benjamin M, Craik FIM (1995) Memory for context and its use in item memory: comparisons of younger and older persons. Psychology and Aging 10: 284–93.

Nicholas M, Obler L, Albert M, Goodglass H (1985) Lexical retrieval in healthy aging. Cortex 21: 595–606.

Obler LK (1980) Narrative discourse style in the elderly. In Obler LK, Albert ML, (Eds) Language and Communication in the Elderly. Lexington, MA: DC Heath and Co.

Obler L, Albert M (1981) Language and aging: a neurobiological analysis. In Beasley D, Davis G, (Eds) Aging: Communication Processes and Disorders. New York: Grune Stratton.

Pratt MW, Boyes C, Robins S, Manchester J (1989) Telling tales: aging, working memory, and the narrative cohesion of storytellers. Developmental Psychology 25: 628–35.

Pratt MW, Robins SL (1991) That's the way it was: age differences in the structure and quality of adults' personal narratives. Discourse Processes 14: 73–85.

Radvansky GA, Curiel JM (1998) Narrative comprehension and aging: the fate of completed goal information. Psychology and Aging 13: 69–79.

Ryan EB, Hummert ML, Boich LH (1995) Communication predicaments of aging: patronizing behavior toward older adults. Journal of Language and Social Psychology 14: 144–66.

Salthouse TA (1996) The processing-speed theory of adult age differences in cognition. Psychological Review 3: 403–28.

Schweich M, van der Linden M, Bredart S, Bruyer R, Nelles B, Schils JP (1992) Daily life difficulties in person recognition reported by young and elderly subjects. Applied Cognitive Psychology 6: 161–72.

Shaner JL (1996) Painful self-disclosures of older adults: judgments of perceived motivations and discloser characteristics. Unpublished doctoral dissertation. Department of Communication Studies, University of Kansas: Lawrence, KS.

Soederberg Miller LM, Stine-Morrow EAL (1998) Aging and the effects of knowledge on on-line reading strategies. Journal of Gerontology: Psychological Sciences 53B: 223–33.

Sommers MS (1996) The structural organization of the mental lexicon and its contribution to age-related declines in spoken-word recognition. Psychology and Aging 11: 333-341.

Stanhope N, Cohen G (1993) Retrieval of proper names: testing the models. British Journal of Psychology 84: 51–65.

Stern C, Prather P, Swinney D, Zurif EB (1991) The time course of automatic lexical access and aging. Brain and Language 40: 359–72.

Stine EAL (1990) On-line processing of written text by younger and older adults. Psychology and Aging 5: 68–78.

Stine EAL, Cheung H, Henderson D (1995) Adult age differences in the on-line processing of new concepts in discourse. Aging and Cognition 2: 1–18.

Stine EAL, Soederberg L, Morrow W (1996) Language and discourse processing in adulthood. In Blanchard-Fields F, (Ed) Perspectives on Cognition in Adulthood. New York: McGraw-Hill.

Stine EAL, Hindman J (1994) Age differences in reading time allocation for propositionally dense sentences. Aging and Cognition 1: 2–16.

Stine EAL, Wingfield A (1988) Memorability functions as an indicator of qualitative age differences in text recall. Psychology and Aging 3: 179–83.

Stine EAL, Wingfield A (1990) The assessment of qualitative age differences in discourse processing. In Hess TM, (Ed) Aging and Cognition: Knowledge Organization and Utilization. North-Holland: Elsevier Science Publishers.

Stine EAL, Wingfield A, Myers SD (1990) Age differences in processing information from television news: the effects of bisensory augmentation. Journals of Gerontology 45: 1–8.

Stine EAL, Wingfield A, Poon LW (1986) How much and how fast: rapid processing of spoken language in later adulthood. Psychology and Aging 1: 303–11.

Stine-Morrow EAL, Loveless MK, Soederberg LM (1996) Resource allocation in on-line reading by younger and older adults. Psychology and Aging 11: 673–88.

Thompson LA (1995) Encoding and memory for visible speech and gestures: a comparison between young and older adults. Psychology and Aging 10: 215–28.

Tun PA (1989) Age differences in processing expository and narrative text. Journal of Gerontology: Psychological Sciences 44: 9–15.

Ulatowska HK, Cannito MP, Hayashi MM, Fleming SG (1995) Language abilities in the elderly. In Ulatowska HK, (Ed) The Aging Brain: Communication in the Elderly. San Diego: College-Hill.

Valentine T, Brennen T, Bredart S (1996) The Cognitive Psychology of Proper Names. London: Routledge.

Waters GS, Caplan D (1996a) The capacity theory of sentence comprehension: critique of Just and Carpenter (1992). Psychological Review 103: 761–72.

Waters GS, Caplan D (1996b) The measurement of verbal working memory capacity and its relation to reading comprehension. Quarterly Journal of Experimental Psychology 49A: 51–79.

Waters GS, Caplan D (1996c) Processing resource capacity and the comprehension of garden path sentences. Memory and Cognition 24: 342–55.

Wingfield A, Stine EAL (1986) Organizational strategies in immediate recall of rapid speech by young and elderly adults. Experimental Aging Research 12: 79–83.

Young AW, Hay DC, Ellis AW (1985) The faces that launched a thousand slips; everyday difficulties and errors in recognizing people. British Journal of Psychology 76: 495–523.

Zacks RT, Hasher L (1997) Cognitive gerontology and attentional inhibition: a reply to Burke and McDowd. Journal of Gerontology: Psychological Sciences 52B: 274–83.

Zacks RT, Hasher L, Doren B, Hamm V (1987) Encoding and memory of explicit and implicit information. Journal of Gerontology 42: 418–22.

Zelinski E (1988) Integrating information from discourse: do older adults show deficits? In Light L, Burke DM, (Eds) Language, Memory, and Aging. New York: Cambridge University Press.

Zelinski EM, Light LL, Gilewski MJ (1984) Adult age differences in memory for prose: the question of sensitivity to passage structure. Developmental Psychology 20: 1181–92.

CHAPTER 7

Semantic processing in Alzheimer's disease

JANE MAXIM, KAREN BRYAN AND KIM ZABIHI

Introduction

Alzheimer's disease is a progressive neurodegenerative disorder with characteristic clinical and pathological features (Cummings and Khachaturian, 1996) and a life expectancy from diagnosis of seven to ten years. It is the most common form of dementia in Europe and North America, with an incidence of 10% in the population over the age of 65, rising to 20% of the population aged over 80. The diagnosis is most commonly made by excluding other causes of the symptoms and, for this reason, the term 'probable Alzheimer's disease' (pAD) will be used to reflect this uncertainty.

One of the key features of pAD is a semantic deficit, in parallel with relative preservation of other areas of language: syntax, phonology and prosody. This semantic deficit can be heard in the conversations of people with pAD. They produce language fluently but there is often a paucity of specific nouns, an increase in pronouns and generic nouns (e.g. *thing*, *someone*, *that*) and reference is underspecified so that it is difficult, for example, for the listener to understand who or what is the focus of that conversation. On tests of generative naming (also known as word fluency), where the person is asked to produce as many items as possible in one category (e.g. animals, towns) in one minute, people with pAD in the early- to mid-stages of the disease process will produce 5 or 6 items compared to the 15–19 produced by age and education matched older people in the normal population (Troster et al., 1989; Kontiola et al., 1990).

A central question in pAD research has been: is this deficit is due to difficulty in accessing semantic information or is information has been lost from the semantic system. That is, given a postulated unitary system in which semantic information is held, is semantic information still within the semantic system but inaccessible, or has the semantic system itself been destroyed by the disease process? This latter position is usually characterized as a degraded store deficit.

This question is not only of theoretical interest but also has very practical implications for people with pAD and their carers. If words and their meanings are difficult to access but are still represented somewhere in the brain, then it may be possible to find strategies that will help access in conversation. If, on the other hand, semantic information is lost altogether, then such strategies will not help and may even be distressing. Advice to, and intervention with people who have a diagnosis of pAD and their carers could be given more appropriately if the nature of the language and cognitive deficits in AD were better understood.

More cogently, pharmacological intervention now offers some hope of slowing the disease process and may even produce some improvement (Harvey 1999; Lovestone, Graham and Howard 1997). If the semantic system in pAD is being systematically destroyed by the neuropathological process of the disease, then little or no improvement could be expected with this intervention. If, however, the semantic system itself is merely increasingly less accessible and what appears to be destruction is only the system systematically 'shutting down' or, more likely, becoming systematically less able to use appropriate connections, then drug intervention might have significant benefits.

In this chapter we report the findings of our research into the status of the semantic system in people diagnosed with pAD. First, however, we review relevant information about Alzheimer's disease, its causes and effects, and previous research into its implications for semantic aspects of language processing.

Alzheimer's disease and its effects on language

Neuropathology of Alzheimer's disease

What is known about the neurological disease process in pAD? The neuropathological findings in pAD include neuronal loss, neurofibrillary tangles, neuritic plaques and amyloid angiopathy, but there are currently no biological markers of pAD that allow presymptomatic detection or definite diagnosis. Diagnosis is accomplished by the use of exclusion criteria and examination of behavioural, cognitive and language disturbances. One of the most widely used sets of criteria for diagnosis in research is the DSM-IV (American Psychiatric Association, 1994): this defines Alzheimer's disease as a syndrome characterized by the development of multiple cognitive deficits, including memory impairment and at least one of the following cognitive disturbances: aphasia, apraxia, agnosia or a disturbance in executive functioning. The deficits must be sufficiently severe to cause impairment in occupational or social functioning and must represent a decline from a previously higher level of functioning. The Alzheimer's disease syndrome must have a gradual onset and continuing cognitive decline. Other neurological disorders, systemic diseases or substance abuse sufficient to induce dementia must be excluded. The deficits must not occur exclusively during delirium and must not be attributable to major psychiatric disorder such as depression.

pAD may be a single pathological entity which presents in different forms (Hardy, 1992) although recent genetic studies point to a number of aetiologies that eventually lead to the AD syndrome e.g. familial Alzheimer's (Rossor, 1992), early onset (Faber-Langendoen, Morris, Knesevich et al., 1988), late onset (Bondareff, 1994), Alzheimer's disease associated with Down's syndrome (Johanson et al., 1991).

Symptom variation and disease progression

It is now widely recognized that there is variation within the disease entity of pAD, but there is considerable debate as to why this variation occurs and its relationship to the neuropathology affecting brain structures. Schwartz describes this heterogeneity as follows:

> . . . each patient presents a landscape of eroding cognitive and functional capacities, but the landscape contains peaks and valleys. One patient may be seen with particularly severe visuospatial confusion and little language disturbance; another patient may show the reverse. Patients may be 'frontal' to a greater or lesser extent. They may have marked extra-pyramidal motor signs . . . More typically most patients show simultaneous dissolution across several domains.
> Schwartz (1990: 143)

Specific symptoms may be associated with faster rates of decline (Chui, Lyness, Sobel et al., 1992) but whether these symptoms reflect a different biological basis to the disease is not known. Joanette, Ska, Poissant et al. (1992) suggest different profiles of deficits and preserved abilities between individuals may be due to individual differences in (1) brain organization for cognition and (2) normal age-related changes in this organization. pAD may present in global, visual or verbal forms, all of which share some semantic deficits but different profiles of deficits and neuropathology (Martin, Brouwers, Lalonde et al., 1986; Martin, 1987; Becker, Huff, Nebes et al., 1988; Fisher, Rourke, Bieliauskas et al. 1996, 1997). Martin et al. (1986) analysed the performance profiles of 43 people with pAD. While the majority of the group had a profile in which retrieval and use of semantic knowledge and visuo-constructional skills both showed deficits, one subgroup had severely impaired naming skills with relatively preserved visuo-constructional skills, while a further group showed the opposite pattern.

Language processing and disease progression

Language deficits in pAD can be significant in both diagnosis and prognosis. It has been found that prevalence and severity of aphasia correlate with duration of illness (Chenery, Murdoch and Ingram (1996) and that early onset pAD predicts the early development of language problems (Chui, Teng, Henderson et al., 1985). Boller, Becker, Holland et al. (1991) suggest that poor performance on language tests, especially naming tests, may be a better predictor of rapid decline in pAD on initial diagnosis than age or severity of dementia. Early onset pAD (before age 65) is associated with greater language deficits than late onset (Faber-Langendoen et al., 1988; Seltzer and Sherwin, 1983), although some studies dispute this finding (Bayles, 1991). Filley, Kelly and Heaton (1986) also found greater disruption in language processing in early onset pAD but interpreted this disruption as being due to variation in disease progression.

Maxim and Bryan (1996) presented a checklist of functions (language, cognition and personality) showing deficits and spared skills at different stages of the disease which is primarily applicable to late onset pAD (Appendix 1) but this information gives a misleading impression of the disease's progression as homogeneous. Language is usually compromised at all stages of pAD but there is an enormous variation in deficits as well as retained functions amongst individuals in the pAD population. Bayles, Tomoeda and Trosset (1992) provide extensive information on language functions linked to stages of the disease measured on the Global Deterioration Rating Scale (Reisberg, Ferris, de Leon et al., 1982) in comparison to normal age- and education-matched controls. There are excellent overviews of language and cognition in pAD in Kempler (1995) and Nebes (1992).

While earlier work on pAD suggests a homogeneous progressive course of semantic deficit, syntactic deficit and finally phonological deficit, people with pAD are almost as likely to be atypical as typical in their presentation and in the course of the disease. Ska, Joanette, Poissant et al. (1990), for example, found that only just over half of their pAD group conformed to the standard account of disease progression. There is, therefore, a consensus that the language symptomatology in pAD is more heterogeneous than previously described and that it is most useful to investigate the deterioration of specific processes.

The semantic system in pAD

Does the semantic system have a reality? Is it a structure in the brain that can be seen, rather than a system that we conceptualize? What we know from imaging studies of brains is that tasks which activate aspects of the conceptual semantic system show a differentiated picture: depending on the task, different parts of the brain appear to function. In other words, current imaging studies suggest that aspects of meaning and knowing are widely distributed in brain structure.

In order to consider what happens to the semantic system in pAD, a working model of language processing (or at least single word processing) is necessary. This working model is made up of a semantic lexicon, and processes that connect into and out of this semantic lexicon. Semantic representations have to be retrieved and associations made between these representations when processing semantic information. It is just these associative relationships and the semantic processes required to make associations that appear to be particularly difficult for people with pAD.

Warrington and Shallice (1979) set up four criteria that have formed the basis for many studies of the semantic system in pAD. These criteria have been used in attempts to differentiate an access problem from a degraded store deficit:

- **Consistency:** in a degraded store deficit, the inability to identify an item should be consistent over testing sessions as the information is permanently lost. This loss should be apparent for different tasks that require identification of the same item.
- **Depth of processing:** in understanding a concept, the superordinate is accessed first, before other conceptual information. In a degraded store deficit, more specific attribute information should be very difficult, if not impossible, to access.
- **Priming:** in a degraded store deficit, if an item cannot be identified, it should not be possible to prime it.
- **Frequency:** more frequent items have a larger and more redundant underlying representation and are therefore less likely to be lost.

These criteria create an elegant and powerful paradigm which has informed the exploration of semantic processing in pAD. While they have been refined and modified by subsequent research, they are a good point from which to begin to investigate the changes to the semantic system in pAD.

Modelling the semantic system

What factors are prominent in any explanation of the changing semantic system in pAD? We have already identified two central issues (*access* versus *loss*; *semantic* or *visual* processing difficulties) which have been the target of extensive research. A third possibility also exists: studies of *priming* (defined here as requiring online processing) and *cueing* (offline processing) suggest that the deficit in Alzheimer's disease may also be at a lexical level outside the semantic system, i.e. the phonological level or in the connections between the semantic and phonological systems.

These hypotheses about the changing semantic system in pAD have been translated into models which are, in effect, a more formal expression of ideas about the system. Models of single word processing which use a modular structure (boxes and arrow models) with a serial throughput of information flow (see Chapter 1) have been used successfully to describe some of the deficits in pAD. These models are particularly useful when the focus is on the language processing system, rather than on the semantic system alone, because they represent an attempt to give a structure to the system overall. In these models, the semantic (or cognitive) system is represented as one central box, but some researchers have hypothesized that the available data are best explained by two semantic systems which process visual and verbal information separately (Shallice, 1993), while there have also been attempts to reconcile the data in pAD by using parallel data processing or connectionist models (Tippett and Farah, 1994). For example, the Organized Unitary Content Hypothesis (OUCH) put forward by Caramazza, Hillis, Rapp et al. (1990) suggests that a single amodal semantic store can account for all data. Access to a semantic representation within OUCH 'results in the activation of all the relevant semantic predicates' (Caramazza et al., 1990: 177), i.e. perceptual, functional and associative predicates. OUCH assumes privileged access for certain types of stimuli so that, for example, an object has privileged access to this system over the word name for that object because it has direct access to perceptual representations while the word name is just that – a phonological form that has become, over time, associated with those predicates. OUCH therefore predicts that there should be better access to the semantic system through objects rather than words and that this should be apparent in the changing semantic system in pAD. Equally, OUCH postulates that there are privileged relationships among predicates. Functional and structural aspects of an object are predicted to have stronger relationships than would exist between them and category membership.

Tippett and Farah (1994) set out to reconcile the evidence of visual and semantic deficits in a computer simulation study. If quality of visual stimuli and frequency of name are a factor in object naming performance, what type of system would be needed to account for both factors? The study also seeks to explain the fact that phonemic cueing may improve naming performance. This work represents an application to pAD data of an earlier model which focused on category and modality-specific deficits (Farah and McClelland, 1991). Using an interactive parallel distributed processing network, they trained this system to associate visual patterns with semantic and lexical patterns. In such models, activation patterns within sets of highly interconnected units simulate proposed neural networks in the brain. The model proposes three layers: (1) semantic units; (2) name and visual input units; (3) name and visual hidden units that are between semantic and input units. The units within each layer are connected and those within and between layers are bi-directional.

Tippett and Farah found that damage (lesions) to the semantic units caused both visual and semantic errors, while phonemic cues were of benefit, and conclude that

> in an interactive system, each component depends for its normal functioning on the output of other components. Therefore, if one component of the system is damaged, the remaining components will be impaired in their functioning, if only to the extent of being more easily taxed by difficult manipulations such as visual impoverishment. Similarly, if processing in one component is bolstered by additional external input, as in phonemic cueing, this may help a system whose damage is in another component.
> Tippett and Farah (1994: 11)

This study elegantly and convincingly demonstrates that damage to the semantic system alone can produce both types of error patterns (semantic and visual) while also accounting for the benefit given by phonemic cues.

More recently, Lambon Ralph, Patterson and Hodges (1997) have put forward a model of semantic organization called Weighted Overlapping Organized Features (WOOF). WOOF seeks to explain the finding that a small but varying number of specific features appear to be crucial for naming to take place. WOOF is amodal and based on the premiss that the semantic system is shaped by how knowledge is acquired. Because this acquisition path will vary, they argue, the cluster of features for any object will be weighted differentially. This weighting allows predictions to be made about the type of information that will be lost. For objects such as tools, for example, where function and associative relationships are a key part of our knowledge about them, these features would be most important while for birds or animals, sensory features are more crucial. The importance of WOOF is in the explicit predictions about how the weighting might work for different types of names and the inclusion of a developmental perspective.

What makes naming difficult in Alzheimer's disease?

Difficulty in finding words that are appropriate and specific to their context is one of the most noticeable features of pAD but deficits on specific tasks such as picture naming are not always an early feature of the disease process (Bayles et al., 1992; Huff, Corkin and Growden, 1986). Other aspects of lexical semantics, on the other hand, such as word fluency, are often a presenting feature. Dick, Kean and Sands (1989) investigated recall of self-generated words in people with pAD compared to a group of normal elderly and found that the pAD group did not show increased recall for self-generated words as the normal elderly did. The ability to name may also have little relation to disease severity. While Skelton-Robinson and Jones (1984) suggest that severity of object naming failure and overall dementia are highly correlated, Bayles and Trosset (1992) found, in a large group of 102 people with pAD, that disease severity did not correlate well with naming ability and that 60% of the variability in naming performance was not explained by disease severity, age at onset, duration of pAD, gender or family history. They concluded that naming in pAD 'can be argued to have a subcomponent that is not subsumed by overall cognitive ability' (Bayles and Trosset, 1992: 197).

The exploration of naming and the knowledge of concepts related to names has usually been through a selection of the following range of tests:

- object naming;
- picture naming;
- word fluency / word generation;
- word definitions;
- word to picture matching;
- picture to picture matching;
- superordinate category tasks;
- probe questions on semantic features.

While some of these tasks (object/picture naming; word–picture or picture–picture matching) can be mapped on to paths through a single word processing model (Ellis and Young, 1988), some require more complex sentence processing. Complexity can be viewed as either making something more difficult or making it easier. If complexity adds more information to the search for a specific word, it may make the task easier.

However, if the complexity requires information from competing sources to be evaluated and processed before a specific word can be retrieved, it may add to the processing load in a way that makes the task more difficult.

The mechanisms causing a breakdown at the level of semantics are only partially understood but there is evidence that, even in the early stages of the disease, access to the semantic system makes naming difficult (Hodges, Salmon and Butters, 1992; Bayles et al., 1992). As the disease progresses, specific items appear to be lost altogether from what remains of the system (Funnel and Hodges, 1990; Hodges et al., 1992; Lambon Ralph et al., 1997). Despite this evidence of deterioration, the semantic system at a single word level may remain partially intact up to a relatively late stage in the disease process (Schwartz, Marin and Saffran, 1979; Nebes, Boller and Holland, 1986; Bayles et al., 1992). Kempler et al. (1990) evaluated consistency as a factor in naming. Testing repeatedly across the same tasks, they found that some patients were consistently unable to name items, while others were inconsistent in the ability to name.

Word frequency has consistently been found to have a significant impact on naming performance (Howes, 1964; Obler, 1980; Skelton-Robinson and Jones, 1984; Hodges et al., 1992). Funnell and Hodges (1990), using data from a longitudinal single case study, argue that the difficulty may lie outside the semantic system, in access between the semantic system and phonological forms of the word, and that word frequency is a significant factor in naming. In a single-word serial processing model, word frequency is predicted to operate outside the semantic system and is a factor in phonological access. This finding of word frequency effects in pAD suggests that the semantic system may not be the only system to undergo change (but see Tippett and Farah, 1994). The data may present evidence that (1) it is not only the semantic system that is impaired; (2) there may be a subgroup of pAD in which the phonological output lexicon is compromised in some way.

An alternative explanation for the picture and object naming decrements is that people with pAD may misperceive visual specifications of the target. The perceptual specification of the target has been shown to alter the success of naming (Grist and Maxim, 1992). The order of ease of naming is the same as that for older people without Alzheimer's disease: a real object, a coloured line drawing, a black and white line drawing, with equivocal results for coloured drawings versus photographs. People with pAD find that visual degradation of such stimuli causes significant difficulty in naming and that the visual complexity of drawings may lead to naming failure, with those drawings identifiable from a characteristic outline being easier to name than those with a more complex outline

(Grist and Maxim, 1992). However, a number of studies suggest (a) that the numbers of such visual misperceptions are few and the ratio of semantic to visual errors is similar to a matched normal population (Shuttleworth and Huber, 1988), and (b) that there is a small subgroup of people with pAD who do undoubtedly have visuo-perceptual problems, which may influence the outcome in group studies (Martin, 1990). Another explanation lies in an interaction between visual processing and the semantic system. If the semantic representation is difficult to access or is lost, then visual stimuli will be interpreted using information that is accessible (Chertkow and Bub, 1992). People with pAD do produce naming errors that have a relationship with the target, i.e. they may pronounce a category name (*animal* for *horse*), a semantically related name (*chair* for *table*) or even a semantic/visual mix (*worm* for *snake*).Might the semantic system be better represented by a distinction into verbal versus visual systems given the repeated finding that people with pAD perform better on visual tasks? Chertkow and Bub (1990a) found that their pAD group showed a loss of conceptual knowledge for both verbal and picture-based tests and that, again, this loss was item specific. However, a subgroup within their study performed better on picture tests than on word tests for pictures that they could classify. Finally, Nicholas, Obler, Au et al. (1996) suggest that a comparison should be made between naming performance in normal and pAD populations. They found that in both populations, error responses were similar in their semantic relatedness to the target.

Features, functions and category-specific knowledge

Language changes are most apparent at the semantic level in pAD but what happens to the semantic system is, as we have discovered when thinking about naming, not easy to interpret. While there is a reduction in naming ability, there is also a breakdown in the ability to make associations. Four particular aspects of associations are of interest because they provide different types of evidence about the organization of the semantic system:

- *superordinate information*: table – non-living;
- *category knowledge*: table – furniture;
- *specific sensory and perceptual features (properties/attributes)*: table – usually has 4 legs; made of wood;
- *functional associative attributes*: table – used for meals; in the kitchen.

This evidence can also be viewed as a hierarchy of conceptual structure. Warrington and Shallice (1979) predicted that lower levels of this hierarchy would be impaired before higher-level information. Features and functional attributes help to differentiate between members of a category. The semantic feature system may appear to deteriorate with more specific features being lost first: that is, 'there is a bottom-up deterioration in semantic knowledge' (Nebes, 1992: 413). Typically, studies in this area have used tasks that require the person to give information about the item or to answer questions with a specific focus:

Category – Is this a piece of furniture?
Feature attribute – Is this sharp?
Functional attributes –Do you clean your teeth with this?

Some of these methods undoubtedly increase processing load. When Chertkow, Bub and Seidenberg (1989) replicated a study done by Martin and Fedio (1983), with the specific aim of decreasing this load, they found better category knowledge and worse feature/function knowledge, with a correlation between inability to name and to answer questions correctly. Some results may therefore be an artefact of the methods used to test people with pAD, rather than a true representation of the semantic system.

Schwartz, Marin and Saffran (1979), in an early single case study, found evidence of a semantic system with specific feature loss which was accessible through only certain modalities and in which more specific semantic features appeared to be lost before more general semantic features. Their subject was able to name only one out of 70 items but demonstrated by gesture that some of the items were recognized. When subjects were asked to select the correct name from five written words, the percentage of correctly recognized objects went up to more than 50%, with one third of the errors being the semantic distractor item. In a group study, Schwartz, Saffran and Williamson (1981) suggested that underselection of the semantic lexical item was a cause of naming failure in pAD. Given a series of four pictures and asked to identify one target item, subjects had much greater difficulty in selecting the correct item from four items of the same class than in identifying one item from four different semantic classes. While the group had difficulty selecting the correct written word when given the word orally, they could match the spoken word more easily to semantically related items.

Is there evidence against specific feature loss? Bayles et al. (1992) argue that the rate of object naming should decline faster than the ability to make category judgements because object naming requires access to specific attributes. Using a group with different levels of severity in comparison with matched normals, they found that object naming was retained better than category judgement ability. Nebes and Brady (1988) used reaction times on four tasks. Their hypothesis was that reaction times to tasks tapping a feature or function should be slower if this knowledge is difficult to access than those tapping category knowledge. Their results, however, showed that the group were slower on category knowledge tasks.

Studies using large groups of people with pAD have concluded that single word comprehension scores are better than naming scores (see, for example, Bayles et al., 1992). However, when the same items are used both in naming and comprehension tasks, small group studies have found item consistency across both tasks and similar patterns of impairment (Schwartz et al., 1981; Chertkow and Bub, 1990b; Hodges, Salmon and Butters 1992). Hodges et al., and Chertkow and Bub, both used similar methodology for the same target items in all tests. Hodges et al. found a significant relationship between the inability to name specific items and the inability to match the same item in a spoken word to picture matching task. There was evidence of preserved superordinate knowledge on definitions and on category sorting when the categories were grossly different (living versus man-made) but deficits emerged as the distinctions to be made required more semantic processing. The pAD group also showed a significant frequency effect when naming.

Differences in methods of testing may create some conflicting results but the overall trend in findings suggests that there are patterns of deficits. There may also be a need to consider whether the pattern of results in pAD mirrors that of an age-matched non-brain-damaged population. Dick et al. (1980), for example, used the normal ageing paradigm in a study which concluded that people with pAD did not show the same pattern as a group of normal elderly of increased recall for self-generated words over picture naming. If similar patterns of results are found for both normal and abnormal populations, then it is more likely that the disease process is systematically reducing access to the system in some way. While pAD does not cause homogeneous deficits, the symptom clusters can be described as a small series of profiles but the neuropathology of pAD shows considerable differentiation.

Cueing, priming and context: can the semantic system be accessed?

Whitacker (1976) demonstrated that the semantic system in pAD can remain partially intact and accessible under certain conditions even at a late stage in the disease process. Her patient (HCEM) had no useful social language but could repeat. Given a noun phrase which contained a phonemic error, HCEM would correct the phrase when shown the actual object. Some phonemic substitutions created a semantically meaningful word (e.g. *pork* for *fork*, *wooden stable* for *wooden table*) but HCEM still corrected the items. Only when HCEM was shown no object did she repeat exactly what the examiner had said. The ability to make this type of repair involves, at a minimum, recognizing the object by accessing the semantic system and then accessing the correct phonological form, presumably already partially activated.

Priming is an effect that makes use of rapid, automatic (implicit) processes and can be contrasted with cueing, which usually makes use of explicit processes. Cueing taps into the use of metalinguistic or metacognitive skills, that is, the ability to think at a conscious level about the task in hand, while priming functions without this attentional knowledge. People with pAD may be unable to name an object (knife) or suggest a function (eat/cut) but they may show a priming effect. Given a word (*knife*) preceded by a related prime word (*cut*), their ability to judge that there is a relationship between these words is facilitated (made faster or more accurate) by the prime. This priming effect demonstrates that (1) there is access to the semantic system; (2) a semantic representation is available to be accessed.

People with pAD show hyper-priming in lexical decision tasks but not in associative priming. Chertkow et al. (1989) used the term hyper-priming to describe their finding that people with pAD appear to benefit more than normal controls from priming. Semantic priming effects have been observed in pAD but the effectiveness of semantic cueing appears weaker (Nebes et al., 1986; Chertkow and Bub, 1990a; Chertkow et al., 1989; Herlitz, Adolfson, Backman et al.,1991). Indeed, Chertkow and Bub found that semantic cueing was not effective but a semantic priming effect was greater for their pAD group than age-matched controls. In addition, the pAD group showed enhanced priming effects on those items that were semantically degraded compared to those that were not. Chertkow and Bub point out that semantic cueing is an offline process whereas semantic priming is an online phenomenon. If we characterize, albeit extremely crudely, online processing as effortful and non-automatic, and offline processing as automatic and not under conscious control, then there are functional implications. We might hypothesize that people with AD will be able to respond better to contexts that do not require effortful processing and interventions might be best targeted at online processes.

Phonological cueing was found to facilitate picture naming in a longitudinal study by Funnell and Hodges (1990) of a single pAD patient. They suggest that access from semantics to the phonological output lexicon, in which spoken word forms are stored, may be another area of deficit. The patient, Mary, was followed over two years and initially spoke fluently although word finding difficulties and circumlocutions were present. Although single word comprehension declined over two years, her comprehension scores remained much better than her naming scores. On picture-naming tests, her performance declined in line with word frequency and she could not name better when given semantic cues. She could, however, repeat the picture names accurately and read them aloud well but she had difficulty in repeating and reading non-words. This discrepancy between word and non-word repetition suggests that the store of word forms (phonological output lexicon) was intact. Mary showed a word frequency effect for naming and was also consistent in her ability to name or failure to name. She could sometimes name when given a phonemic cue after having failed to name spontaneously, but phonemic cueing became less effective as overall naming scores decreased.

Does context have an effect on phrase or sentence processing? We have already described how attribute or function tasks may be easier for people with pAD than identification of a single word or object. People with pAD may show naming behaviours that may reflect changes to the semantic system. Several studies describe the use of phrases such as *cutting blade*, *hand bell*, *ink pen*, *drinking cup* which are added on to the object name; in other cases object names may be replaced by a phrase which describes an attribute or function of the object. Bayles and Tomoeda (1983), for example, found that over a quarter of incorrect naming responses were correct contexts or functions. Such behaviour suggests that these patients have some ability to monitor and change their language behaviour in context.

One characteristic of language use in pAD is the repeated use of specific words, phrases or even short sentences, either in monologues or in conversational language. Such language use is sometimes perseverative but sometimes words and phrases may be used as markers when other lexical items are not available. Such intrusions or even confabulations may be produced where correct information appears inaccessible (Dalla Barba and Wong, 1992; Dalla Barba, Wong, Parlato et al., 1992). Another important pointer to discourse change in pAD is repair of the errors. Speech errors are naturally occurring phenomena which are present in normal populations. Most of these errors are repaired quickly (within the same clause) via monitoring mechanisms in language processing. McNamara, Obler, Au et al. (1992) found that 24% of speech errors were repaired in their pAD group, compared to a range of 72–92% for a healthy elderly control group. The pAD group used very few single word repairs but relied on adding new syntactic information, suggesting that these monitoring mechanisms are partially intact. Discourse analysis is another form of linguistic analysis that has been used to describe changes in conversational interactions (Hutchinson and Jensen, 1980; Ripich and Terrell, 1988; Ulatowska, North and Macaluso-Haynes, 1981). Findings suggest that people with pAD change their strategies for discourse. While lack of clear referents is a common finding, people with pAD may change the topic of conversation when they cannot respond appropriately in conversation (Hutchinson and Jenson, 1980; Ska and Guenard, 1993). This strategy suggests that in the early- to mid-stages of pAD, some metalinguistic awareness remains.

Semantic processing in pAD across modalities, tasks and time: a research report

So far, the picture of semantic processing in pAD that has emerged is of a deteriorating system with both degradation of information and lack of access contributing to the overall picture. If we modify the methodology commonly used for testing individuals with pAD, does a different picture emerge? The data in this section come from studies that were set up explicitly to explore what is working in the semantic system and whether items that appear to be lost can be accessed (Clifford, 1997; Zabihi, 2000).These studies explore how specific sets of vocabulary items and categories are processed across modalities, tasks and time. In particular, we look at categorical knowledge, unique feature attributes, and cueing, across testing sessions approximately eight months apart.

Given a constrained set of vocabulary items, if representations are still in the semantic system, then searching across different tasks, modalities and at different times will reveal variable accessibility but few, if any, lost items. Specifically, we should expect that:

* input and output tasks would show different performance levels;
* naming performance over time would show item inconsistency;
* cueing would allow unnamed items to be accessed;
* cueing success would be variable over time and across items;
* access should be demonstrable as overall severity increases;
* access to category knowledge would not be easier than access to attribute knowledge.

A cognitive and language screening battery was assembled to provide information on the subjects' overall performance in cognition, language-related cognitive performance and specific semantic performance. The cognitive and language-related cognitive battery consisted of:

* Global Deterioration Scale for Assessment of Primary Degenerative Dementia (GDS: Reisberg et al., 1982);
* Clifton Assessment Procedures for the Elderly (CAPE: Pattie, 1981; survey version);

- The Visual Object and Space Perception Battery (VOSP: Warrington and James, 1990; shape detection and dot counting subtests);
- The National Adult Reading Test (NART: Nelson, 1982; shortened version: Beardsall and Brayne, 1990)
- The Set Test (Isaacs and Akhtar, 1972; generative naming tasks in four semantic categories: animals, colours, fruits and towns);
- The Pyramids and Palm Trees Test (Howard and Patterson, 1992; three picture version);
- The British Picture Vocabulary Scales (BPVS: Dunn, Dunn, Whetton et al., 1982)

A set of experimental tasks to examine specific semantic functioning was constructed, using the same pool of vocabulary items and categories across tasks (Zabihi 2000). The test stimuli were black and white line drawings and printed words. The categories were 15 of the most common semantic categories in Battig and Montague (1969) and the standardized line drawings were mainly taken from Snodgrass and Vanderwart (1980). The tasks within the semantic test battery were as follows.

- *Recognition of nouns by semantic category*: the Picture and Written word versions were used. Subjects were asked to point to three pictures that belonged to the same semantic category, out of five categories.
- *Recognition of nouns by unique feature attribute*: the Picture and Written word versions were used. Subjects were asked to recognize pictures and words by unique feature attribute from a target picture/word and four distractors of the following type: visual, close semantic, distant semantic and unrelated.
- *Picture-naming of object pictures*: items from the vocabulary pool were used.
- *Generative naming*: there were 15 semantic categories, drawn from semantic categories used in other tests: 6 living and 9 non-living object categories.

Eight people with pAD were compared to 20 normal healthy older people matched for age, education and IQ, this latter group being defined as people who were maintaining themselves in their own homes and who had no diagnosed neurological or psychiatric disease. The pAD subjects had a mean age of 79.4 years (range 70–91) and were estimated as between 2 and 4 years post onset. On the Global Deterioration Scale, 4 fell into GDS stage 2/3 and 4 into GDS Stage 4–5. Initial testing on both the cognitive and semantic tasks indicated that the pAD subjects were performing at a significantly lower level than the control subjects. Comparison between those with pAD scoring 2/3 compared to those scoring 4/5 on GDS also showed significant differences between these two levels of severity on cognitive and language tasks, demonstrating that the semantic screening battery was sensitive to change in the semantic processing system. A comparison of the mean scores of the pAD subjects on the cognitive and language tasks in the initial test, and the re-test eight months later indicated that there was no significant deterioration of the pAD subjects' mean performance on each cognitive or language task over the eight month period. Given the long course of Alzheimer's disease (7–10 years), this finding is not unexpected.

How well did the pAD group perform on the language tasks compared to the controls?

The performance of pAD subjects on tasks that required access to the semantic system was then analysed as a percentage of the control mean to establish an overall picture of the nature and severity of impairment (Table 1). Generative naming abilities (55%) and the recognition by category tasks (picture recognition by category = 49%; word recognition by category = 60%) were most significantly impaired. On the recognition by unique attribute tasks (picture recognition of attribute and word recognition of attribute) the pAD group performed at over 90% of the control mean.

Table 1. Mean scores on semantic tests for the pAD group expressed as a percentage of control mean.

Task	Mean score for pAD subjects	Percentage of control mean
Generative naming 1	25	46.9
Generative naming 3	29	48
Picture recognition by category	6.6/30	48.7
Generative naming 2	33.6	53
Word recognition by category	8.7/30	60
Naming	44.8/60	76.5
Picture recognition by attribute	27.3/30	91
Word recognition by attribute	27.5/30	92

Does comparison across different tasks and modalities reveal variable access to the vocabulary set?

Picture-naming capacities were relatively preserved (76.5% of control mean) in comparison to generative naming capacities (55% of control mean) of the same categories of items (Table 2). Both GDS stage 2–3 and GDS stage 4–5 groups showed the same pattern of better confrontation naming than generative naming. While this result does reveal variable access to items across two types of name production task, the demands of these two tasks are different. *Picture-naming* requires identification of a single picture, subsequent access to the semantic system and the phonological output lexicon before a name is produced. It can be argued that generative naming is more complex, requiring identification of category knowledge through a search of the semantic system for category members.

The mean scores of the pAD subjects on the recognition tasks as a percentage of the control mean (Table 1), shows that performance in picture and word recognition by unique attribute was higher than performance on picture and word recognition by category. In the unique attribute recognition tasks, the subjects scored at a 92% and 90% level respectively of the control mean in comparison to the category tasks where the subjects scored at a 60% and 48% level of the control mean respectively. If category information has to be accessed first, then category tasks should be easier than attribute tasks, but this is not so here. For both severity levels, the performance of the GDS stage 2–3 and 4–5 groups showed better preservation for recognition by unique attribute in comparison to recognition by category (Table 2).

Table 2. Performance of the GDS stage 2–3 and 4–5 pAD groups on tests of recognition by unique attribute and recognition by category.

Task	GDS Stage 2–3 Group		GDS Stage 4–5 Group	
	Mean Score n=30	Percentage of Control Mean	Mean Score n=30	Percentage of Control Mean
Picture Attribute	29.5	98	25	83
Word Attribute	29.5	97.5	21	76
Picture Category	11	76	7.5	52
Word Category	9.5	70	4.75	36

Could this difference be due to processing load, rather than variable access? In the unique attribute task, subjects were given a card on which there were five words or pictures. They were then given the instruction: 'Show me the one which . . .', followed by the unique attribute of the target item. For example, the unique attribute for 'peacock' was 'proud of its plumage'. This required understanding the attribute, followed by a visual search before identification. In the category recognition task, the subjects were instructed: 'Show me the three objects which go together.'

This required a visual search and deletion of non-congruent items. Because the tasks require such different processes, it is hard to argue that one is more difficult than the other.

If we assume that the category task is, in some sense, more difficult, then we might expect that both the picture and written forms would show similar patterns of deficit; however, for half the group there are differences of 3 or more errors out of 30 between these two conditions. If we compare picture and word unique attribute conditions, again there is little consistency between performance on the same task but using different modalities (Table 3).

Table 3. Unique attribute conditions and category conditions across picture and word modalities.

Subject	Category picture v Category word	Category picture v Attribute picture	Category word v Attribute word	Attribute picture v Attribute word
1	=	=	=	=
2	=	<	<	=
3	<	=	<	=
4	=	<	<	=
5	>	=	=	>
6	<	=	<	>
7	=	<	<	=
8	<	=	<	=

= Performance is equivalent on both tasks.
< >Performance shows lesser (<) or greater (>) deficits on first task.

How did people with pAD perform on other tests that require recognition?

On the BPVS test of single spoken word to picture comprehension, the pAD group had a mean score of 75% of the controls. A similar mean score was obtained on the Pyramids and Palm Trees test (76% and 74% in Table 4), a test of conceptual or visual semantics. The pAD mean scores across visual perceptual tasks are close to the control mean.

Does cueing allow unnamed items to be accessed?

All pAD subjects were able to benefit from cueing, with all but one subject benefiting from both semantic and phonemic cues. Semantic cues (for the unique attribute: e.g. 'a man's best friend' for *dog*) were given after 15 seconds had been allowed for naming. If the semantic cue did not elicit the name, a phonemic cue was given (usually the first syllable in polysyllabic words, the first consonant and vowel or initial vowel in monosyllabic words).The number of items named after cues was calculated as a percentage of the number of items unable to be named on first response (Table 5).

Table 4. Cognitive and language-related recognition tasks.

	CAPE	VOSP 1	VOSP 2	BPVS	Pyramids and Palm Trees
	n=12	n=10	n=20	n=32	n=30
Controls	11.6	9.9	20	29.9	29.8
pAD Test 1	6.5 (56%)	8.5 (85%)	17.9 (90%)	22.7 (76%)	22.6 (76%)
pAD Test 2	5.9 (51%)	9 (90%)	16.6 (83%)	21.4 (74%)	22 (74%)

Table 5. Naming and cueing.

Subject	Correct names n=60	Unable to name	Name with semantic cue	Name with phonemic cue	% success with cue	Unnamed
F3	42	18	11	5	89	2
F2	53	7	3	3	86	1
F5	49	11	8	1	82	2
F8	50	10	7	1	80	2
F4	33	27	13	7	75	7
F7	37	23	9	7	69	7
F1	49	11	7	0	64	4
F6	38	22	6	2	36	14

A high percentage (mean 73.25%) of the items that the pAD subjects were unable to name spontaneously were named following a semantic or phonemic cue. There is also some relationship between the success of naming and success of cueing (Table 5). One subject (F4) had the lowest spontaneous naming score (33) but cueing allowed a further 20 items to be named. This subject also had low scores on VOSP and other tests using pictures, with higher scores on tests using words, suggesting a specific visual perceptual deficit for pictures. Cueing presumably allowed enough access to the semantic system, perhaps via an information cascade. The success of phonemic cues after time when semantic cues have failed to elicit the word is somewhat problematic. In Table 5, it is clear that, for most subjects, semantic cues elicited names better than phonemic cues. However, it should be noted that phonemic cues were last in the cueing process and the result might have been different if the order of cueing had been reversed. Phonemic cues may have an effect because (a) the person is in a tip of the tongue state; (b) they allow partially accessed semantic information to be fully accessed; or (c) there may be a frequency effect for the phonemic information given for some words (*cat*, *bat*).

Was consistency a factor in either naming ability or naming failure?

In the 8 or more month interval between testing, the number of items that were named after cueing increased from 66% to 75%. This improvement was unexpected. In order to look at consistency in naming failure, the number of items in successive tests that each subject was unable to name, after a phonemic cue and/or a semantic cue, was compared across the two tests (Table 6). Half the subjects were consistently unable to name a very small number of items in successive tests after a phonemic and/or semantic cue. The remaining subjects showed an inconsistent inability to name items across the testing situations. Could the subjects identify these consistently unnamed items? Each subject could identify the objects by their attribute in the picture recognition by attribute task. Similarly, three of the four subjects were able to select semantic categories of the items they consistently were unable to recall. Only one subject (F8) showed consistency across tasks for a small number of items.

Table 6. Picture naming consistency.

Subject	Number of items unnamed after tests	Number of items consistently unable to name after cues		Number of items unnamed after cues
		Test 1	Test 2	
S1	2	1	1	1
S2	2	1	0	0
S3	3	0	0	0
S4	7	1	2	2
S5	5	1	0	0
S6	8	5	2	1
S8	4	2	2	1

The items produced in the Generative Naming Tasks were then analysed to establish whether items were produced consistently across testings. The percentage of items named in the second test that were not named in the initial task was calculated for each test (Table 7). Between 15% and 68% of items named in the second testing were different from items named in the first testing, even though the overall number of items for each subject across testings decreased.

Table 7. Percentage of different items produced in generative naming.

Subject	Mean percentage
S4	68
S3	57
S5	55.1
S6	55.6
S8	55.5
S2	33.1
S1	17.1

What conclusions can we draw from these findings?

The semantic system, at least in this group of mild to moderate impaired people with pAD, appears inaccessible rather than degraded. There is inconsistency in:

- input versus output tasks;
- picture versus word recognition tasks;
- generative naming across time-modality differences.

In addition, misnamings were largely semantic, rather than visual, and most of the pAD group responded to cueing, with semantic cueing producing a larger number of target names. For each individual, there is evidence of access problems, but only one subject exhibited item consistency. Could these findings be due to a frequency effect? It is the case that the items chosen were of varying frequencies, and yet access could be demonstrated for almost all items under one condition; consequently, frequency is less likely to explain performance.

Could severity have been a factor in this result? The GDS scale goes up to a severity of 7, so that the four subjects whose GDS rating was 4–5 were only in the moderate to severe range. People with pAD become increasingly unable to co-operate with testing procedures that require initiation of action. Even at GDS 4–5, these subjects were markedly more likely to give 'don't know' responses or not to respond. Yet even at this stage in the disease process, we could demonstrate access to the representations for some items. However, there appears to be some evidence that accessing becomes increasingly more difficult as severity develops, and we would argue that the deficit is one in which accessing becomes systematically more difficult.

What are the implications of current research for people with pAD?

1. Undoubtedly there is progressive and widespread damage to cortical tissue in pAD and it would be foolish to argue with the terminal loss to cognitive and language function that this damage must bring about. However, the research reviewed here suggests that access to the semantic system is a major component in the semantic impairment in pAD and that even at later stages in the disease process, access to the semantic system is possible, even if the system is degraded.

2. People with pAD have heterogeneous profiles which make it important to consider the cognitive and language skills of the individual with pAD. Impairment in cognitive functions can have an impact on performance in language assessments. This was demonstrated by one subject whose visual difficulties lowered scores on the picture-naming test. Similarly, this may work in reverse where specific semantic processing difficulties may make it difficult to respond to questions in the CAPE survey.

3. Although some studies have shown close correspondence between input and output tests, this is not always the case. Mary (Funnell and Hodges, 1990), for example, demonstrated relatively preserved understanding of concepts compared with her ability to produce names.

4. The rate of deterioration may be uneven and, particularly in the early stages of the disease, slow. This has implications for pharmacological intervention and suggests that early diagnosis should be the norm, rather than the exception.

5. In clinical management, it is important to establish whether the difficulties are likely to be accounted for by an access disorder or by loss of items and whether visuo-perceptual difficulties are present. If cueing techniques are effective in enhancing naming performance on testing, then semantic facilitation needs to be built into everyday interaction so that communication can be enhanced for as long as possible.

6. The pAD population might, we hypothesize, begin the process of semantic deterioration with an access problem. At a later stage, there may be both access and loss of semantic representations, followed finally by a late stage where it is probably not possible to demonstrate either process by conventional testing but degradation of the semantic system would be more likely.

References

American Psychiatric Association (1994) Diagnostic and Statistical Manual of Mental Disorders (4th edition) Washington DC: American Psychiatric Association.

Battig WF, Montague WE (1969) Category norms for verbal items in 56 categories. Journal of Experimental Psychology 80: 1–46.

Bayles KA (1991) Age at onset of Alzheimer's disease: relation to language dysfunction. Archives of Neurology 48(2): 155–59.

Bayles KA (1992) Arizona Battery of Communication in Dementia. Tucson, AZ: Communication Skills Builders.

Bayles KA, Tomoeda CK (1983) Confrontation naming impairment in dementia. Brain and Language 19: 98–114.

Bayles KA, Tomoeda CK, Trosset MW (1992) Relation of linguistic communication abilities of Alzheimer's patients to stage of disease. Brain and Language 42: 454–72.

Bayles KA, Trosset MW, (1992) Confrontation naming in Alzheimer's patients: relation to disease severity. Psychology and Aging 7(2): 197–203.

Beardsall L, Brayne C (1990) Estimation of verbal intelligence in an elderly community: a prediction analysis using a shortened NART. British Journal of Clinical Psychology 29: 83–90.

Becker JT, Huff J, Nebes RD, Holland A, Boller F (1988) Neuropsychological function in Alzheimer's disease: patterns of impairment and rates of progression. Archives of Neurology 45: 263–68.

Boller F, Becker JT, Holland AL, Forbes MM, Hood PC, McCougle-Gibson KC (1991) Predictors of decline in Alzheimer's disease.

Bondareff W (1994) Subtypes of Alzheimer's Disease. In Burns A and Levy R (eds). Dementia. London: Chapman and Hall.

Bryan K, Maxim J, (Eds) (1996) Communication Disability and the Psychiatry of Old Age. London: Whurr.

Caramazza A, Hillis AE, Rapp BC, Romani C (1990) The multiple semantics hypothesis: multiple confusions? Cognitive Neuropsychology 7: 161–89.

Chenery HJ, Ingram JCL, Murdoch B (1998) The resolution of lexical ambiguity with reference to context in dementia of the Alzheimer's type. International Journal of Language and Communication Disorders 33(4): 393–412.

Chenery HJ, Murdoch B, Ingram JCL (1996) An investigation of confrontation naming performance in Alzheimer's disease as a function of disease severity. Aphasiology 10(5): 423–41.

Chertkow H, Bub D (1990a) Semantic memory loss in dementia of Alzheimer's type: what do various measures measure? Brain 113: 397–417.

Chertkow H, Bub D (1990b) Semantic memory loss in Alzheimer-type dementia. In Schwartz MF, (Ed) Modular Deficits in Alzheimer-type Dementia. Cambridge, MA: MIT Press. pp 207–44.

Chertkow H, Bub D (1992) Constraining theories of semantic memory processing: evidence from dementia. Cognitive Neuropsychology 9: 327–65.

Chertkow H, Bub D, Seidenberg M (1989) Priming and semantic memory loss in Alzheimer's disease. Brain and Language 36: 420–46.

Chui HC, Lyness S, Sobel E, Schneider LS (1992) Prognostic implications of symptomatic behaviours in AD. In Florette F, Khachaturian Z, Poncet M, Christen Y, (Eds) Heterogeneity of Alzheimer's Disease. Berlin: Springer.

Chui HC, Teng EL, Henderson VW, Moy AC (1985) Clinical subtypes of dementia of the Alzheimer type. Neurology 35: 1544–50.

Clifford S (1997) An investigation into the nature of language decline in Alzheimer's disease. Unpublished MSc thesis. University College, London.

Cummings JL, Khachaturian Z (1996) Definitions and diagnostic criteria. In Gauthier S, (Ed) Clinical Diagnosis and Management of Alzheimer's Disease. London: Dunitz. pp 3–16.

Dalla Barba G, Wong C (1992) Encoding specificity and confabulation in Alzheimer's disease and amnesia. Journal of Clinical and Experimental Neuropsychology 3: 378–92.

Dalla Barba G, Wong C, Parlato V, Boller F (1992) Encoding specificity, anosagnosia and confabulation in Alzheimer's disease and depression. Neurobiology of Aging 13: 4–5.

Dick MB, Kean M-L, Sands D (1989) Memory for internally generated words in Alzheimer-type dementia: breakdown in encoding and semantic memory. Brain and Cognition 9: 88–108.

Dunn MD, Dunn LM, Whetton C, Pintillie D (1982) British Picture Vocabulary Scale. Windsor: NFER-Nelson Publishing Co Ltd.

Ellis AW, Young AW (1988) Human Cognitive Neuropsychology. Hove and London: Lawrence Erlbaum Associates.

Faber-Langendoen K, Morris JC, Knesevich JW, LaBarge E, Miller JP, Berg L (1988) Aphasia in senile dementia of the Alzheimer type. Annual Neurology 23: 365–70.

Farah MJ, McClelland JL (1991) A computational model of semantic memory impairment; modality specificity and emergent category specificity. Journal of Experimental Psychology: General 120: 339–57.

Filley CM, Kelly J, Heaton RK (1986) Neuropsychologic features of early and late onset Alzheimer's disease. Archives of Neurology 43: 574–76.

Fisher NJ, Rourke BP, Bieliauskas LA, Giordani B, Berent S, Foster NL (1996) Neuropsychological subgroups of patients with Alzheimer's disease. Journal of Clinical and Experimental Psychology 18: 349–70.

Fisher NJ, Rourke BP, Bieliauskas LA, Giordani B, Berent S, Foster NL (1997) Unmasking the heterogeneity of Alzheimer's disease: case studies of individuals from distinct neuropsychological subgroups. Journal of Clinical and Experimental Psychology 19: 713–54.

Funnell E, Hodges J (1990) Progressive loss of access to spoken word forms in a case of Alzheimer's disease. Proceedings of the Royal Society of London B243: 173–79.

Grist E, Maxim J (1992) Confrontation naming in the elderly: the Build–up Picture Test as an aid to differentiating normals from subjects with dementia. European Journal of Disorders of Communication 27: 197–207.

Hardy J (1992) Alzheimer's disease: many aetologies; one pathogenesis. In: Florette F, Khachaturian Z, Poncet M, Christen Y (eds) Heterogeneity of Alzheimer's Disease. Berlin: Springer-Verlag.

Harvey RJ (1999) A review and commentary on a sample of 15 UK guidelines for the drug treatment of Alzheimer's Disease. International Journal of Geriatric Psychiatry 14: 249–256.

Herlitz A, Adolfson R, Backman L, Wilson L-G (1991) Cue utilization following different forms of encoding in mildly moderately and severely demented patients with Alzheimer's disease. Brain and Cognition 15: 119–30.

Hodges JR, Salmon DP, Butters N (1992) Semantic memory impairment in Alzheimer's disease: failure of access or degraded knowledge? Neuropsychologia 30(4): 301–14.

Howard D, Patterson K (1992) The Pyramids and Palm Trees Test. Bury St Edmunds: Thames Valley Test Company.

Howes D (1964) Application of the word frequency concept to aphasia. In de Rueck AVS, O'Connor M, (Eds) Disorders of Language. Ciba Foundation Symposium. London: Churchill.

Huff FJ, Corkin S, Growden JH (1986) Semantic impairment and anomia in Alzheimer's disease. Brain and Language 28: 235–49.

Hutchinson JM, Jensen M (1980) A pragmatic evaluation of discourse communication in normal and senile elderly in a nursing home. In Obler LK, Albert ML, (Eds) Language and Communication in the Elderly. Lexington, MA: DC Heath and Co.

Isaacs B, Akhtar AJ (1972) The Set Test: a rapid test of mental function in old people. Age and Ageing 1: 222–26.

Joanette Y, Ska B, Poissant A, Beland R (1992) Neuropsychological aspects of Alzheimer's disease: evidence for inter- and intra-function heterogeneity. In Florette F, Khachaturian Z, Poncet M, Christen Y, (Eds) Heterogeneity of Alzheimer's Disease. Berlin: Springer.

Johanson A, Gustafson L, Brun A, Risberg J, Rosen I, Tideman E (1991) A longitudinal study of dementia of Alzheimer type in Down's syndrome. Dementia 1(2): 159–68.

Kempler D, Anderson E, Hunt M, Henderson V (1990) Linguistic and attentional contributions to anomia in Alzheimer's Disease. Journal of Clinical and Experimental Neuropsychology 12: 398–406.

Kempler D (1995) Language changes in dementia of the Alzheimer type. In Lubinski R, (Ed) Dementia and Communication. California: Singular Publishing Group. pp 98–114.

Kontiola P, Laaksoner R, Sulkawa R, Erkinjunsi T (1990) Pattern of language impairment in Alzheimer's disease and multi–infarct dementia. Brain and Language 38: 364–83.

Lambon Ralph MA, Patterson K, Hodges JR (1997) The relationship between naming and semantic knowledge for different categories in dementia of Alzheimer's type. Neuropsychologia 35(9).

Lovestone S, Graham N, Howard RR (1997) Guidelines on drug treatment for Alzheimer's Disease. Lancet 350/9073: 232–233.

Martin A (1987) Representations of semantic and spatial knowledge in Alzheimer's patients: implications for models of preserved learning in amnesia. Journal of Clinical and Experimental Neuropsychology 9: 121–224.

Martin A (1990) Neuropathology of Alzheimer's disease: the case for subgroups. In Schwartz MF, (Ed) Modular Deficits in Alzheimer-type Dementia. Cambridge, MA: MIT Press. pp 144–78.

Martin A, Brouwers P, Lalonde F, Cox C, Teleska P, Fedio P, Forster NL, Chase TN (1986) Towards a behavioural typology of Alzheimer's patients. Journal of Clinical and Experimental Neuropsychology.

Martin A, Fedio P (1983) Word production and comprehension in Alzheimer's disease: the breakdown of semantic knowledge. Brain and Language 34: 262–78.

Maxim J, Bryan K (1996) Language, cognition and communication in the older mentally infirm. In: Bryan K, Maxim J (eds) Communication Disability and the Psychiatry of Old Age. London: Whurr, p. 38–79.

McNamara P, Obler LK, Au R, Durso R, Albert ML (1992) Speech monitoring skills in Alzheimer's disease, Parkinson's disease and normal ageing. Brain and Language 42: 38–51.

Nebes RD (1992) Cognitive dysfunction in Alzheimer's disease. In Craik FIM, Salthouse TA, (Eds) The Handbook of Aging and Cognition. Hillsdale, NJ: Lawrence Erlbaum Associates. pp 373–448.

Nebes RD, Boller F, Holland A (1986) Use of semantic context by patients with Alzheimer's disease, Psychology and Ageing 1: 261–69.

Nebes RD, Brady CB (1988) Integrity of semantic fields in Alzheimer's disease. Cortex 24: 291–300.

Nelson (1982) National Adult Reading Test (NART).

Nicholas M, Obler LK, Au R, Albert ML (1996) On the nature of naming errors in aging and dementia: a study of semantic relatedness. Brain and Language 54(2): 184–95.

Obler LK (1980) Narrative discourse style in the elderly. In Obler L, Albert M, (Eds) Language and Communication in the Elderly. Lexington, MA: DC Heath and Co.

Pattie AH (1981) A survey version of the Clifton Assessment Procedures for the Elderly (CAPE). British Journal of Clinical Psychology 20: 173–78.

Reisberg B, Ferris SM, de Leon M, Crook T (1982) The global deterioration scale for assessment of primary degenerative dementia. American Journal of Psychiatry 139: 1136–39.

Ripich DN, Terrell BY (1988) Patterns of discourse cohesion in Alzheimer's disease. Journal of Speech and Hearing Disorders 53: 8–15.

Rossor MN, Kennedy AM, Newman SK (1992) Heterogeneity in familial Alzheimer's disease. In Florette F, Khachaturian Z, Poncet M, Christen Y, (Eds) Heterogeneity of Alzheimer's Disease. Berlin: Springer.

Schwartz MF (1990) Modular Deficits in Alzheimer-type Dementia. Cambridge, MA: MIT-Bradford.

Schwartz MF, Marin OS, Saffran EM (1979) Dissociation of language function in dementia: a case study. Brain and Language 7: 277–306.

Schwartz MF, Saffran EM, Williamson S (1981) The breakdown of lexicon in Alzheimer's dementia. Paper given at Linguistic Society of America 56th Annual Meeting: New York, USA.

Seltzer B, Sherwin I (1983) A comparison of clinical features in early and late onset primary degenerative dementia: one entity or two? Archives of Neurology 40: 143–46.

Shallice T (1979) Case-study approach in neuropsychological research. Journal of Clinical Neuropsychology 1: 183–211.

Shallice T (1993) Multiple semantics: whose confusions? Cognitive Neuropsychology 10(3): 251–61.

Shuttleworth EC, Huber S J (1988) The naming disorder of dementia of Alzheimer type. Brain and Language 34: 222–34.

Ska B, Guenard D (1993) Narrative schema in dementia of the Alzheimer's type. In Brownell HH, Joanette Y, (Eds) Narrative Discourse in Neurologically Impaired and Normal Aging Adults. San Diego, CA: Singular Publishing Group. pp 299–316.

Ska B, Joanette Y, Poissant A, Beland R, Lecours AR (1990) Language disorders in dementia of the Alzheimer type: contrastive patterns from a multiple single case study. Abstract of the Academy of Aphasia 28th Annual Meeting, Oct: Baltimore, USA. pp 21–23.

Skelton-Robinson M, Jones S (1984) Nominal dysphasia and the severity of senile dementia. British Journal of Psychiatry 145: 168–71.

Snodgrass JG, Vanderwart M (1980) A standardised set of 260 pictures: norms for name agreement, familiarity, and visual complexity. Journal of Experimental Psychology: General 6: 174–215.

Tippett LJ, Farah MJ (1994) A computational model of naming in Alzheimer's disease: unitary or multiple impairments? Neuropsychology 8(1): 3–13.

Troster AI, Salmon DP, McCullough D, Butters N (1989) A comparison of the category fluency deficits associated with Alzheimer's and Huntingdon's disease. Brain and Language 37: 500–13.

Ulatowska H, North AJ, Macaluso-Haynes S (1981) Production of narrative and procedural discourse in aphasia. Brain and Language 13: 345–71.

Warrington EK, James M (1990) VOSP: Visual Perception and Space Perception Battery. Bury St Edmunds: Thames Valley Test Company.

Warrington EK, Shallice T (1979) Semantic access dyslexia. Brain 102: 43–63.

Whitacker H (1976) A case of the isolation of the language function. In Whitacker H, Whitacker HA, (Eds) Studies in Neurolinguistics 2. New York: Academic Press.

Zabihi K (2000) A comparative investigation into knowledge of object attributes of name unique function and category membership in healthy elders and old people with Alzheimer-type dementia. Unpublished MPhil thesis. University College, London.

Appendix

Checklist of functions for late-onset Alzheimer's disease (Maxim and Bryan 1996)

EARLY-STAGE ALZHEIMER'S DISEASE

Language

- Low frequency word finding impairment
- Circumlocution in conversation
- Word fluency impaired
- Composite picture description incomplete
- Poor repetition of BDAE low frequency sentences
- Utterance completion poor in conversation
- Auditory and written complex sentence comprehension impaired
- Single word recognition maintained

Cognition

- Episodic memory impaired
- Specific autobiographical memory impaired
- Time orientation impaired
- Impaired famous faces naming
- Attention impaired
- Time orientation impaired

Personality

- Change of affect
- Avoidance/denial strategies
- Increased anxiety
- Depression

MID-STAGE ALZHEIMER'S DISEASE

Language

- Naming deficits on high frequency items
- Semantic paraphasias
- Reference deficit in pronoun use
- Errors in complex sentence production
- Occasional phonemic paraphasias
- Decrease in semantic cuing response
- Sentence reading aloud poor
- Single regular word reading aloud retained
- Decreased use of gesture
- Poor repetition of BDAE high frequency sentences
- Single word recognition impairment
- Simple sentence comprehension impairments

Cognition

- Impaired working memory
- Decreased knowledge of current events
- Ideational perseveration
- Time and place orientation impaired
- Calculation deficits
- Visuo-spatial and perceptual deficits

Other

- Wandering and exit seeking behaviour
- Increasing apathy
- Sleep disturbance
- Assistance needed in activities of daily living

LATE-STAGE ALZHEIMER'S DISEASE

Language

- Language initiation decreased/ceases
- Noun use non-specific/non-existent
- Phonemic paraphasias on repetition
- Stereotypical utterances
- Verbal perseverations
- Echolalia possible
- No use of gesture

Cognition

- Time, place and person disorientation
- Face recognition poor

Other

- Dependent for activities of daily living
- Poor eye contact
- Inappropriate social behaviour
- Poor mobility
- Purposeless motor movements
- Incontinence
- Feeding and swallowing disorder

CHAPTER 8

Semantic dementia: assessment and management

JULIE S. SNOWDEN AND HELEN GRIFFITHS

Clinical overview

Semantic dementia designates a distinct clinical syndrome that results from focal degenerative disease of the temporal lobes (Breedin, Saffran and Coslett, 1994; Hodges, Patterson, Oxbury et al., 1992; Snowden, Goulding and Neary, 1989; Snowden, Neary and Mann, 1996b). The disorder is characterized by a progressive and yet selective loss of semantic knowledge. A central component of the disorder is loss of word meaning, so the patient can no longer name or understand the meaning of words, yet the semantic impairment is not confined to the verbal domain. It may encompass all sensory modalities, so that patients have difficulty recognizing the identity of familiar faces and objects, of non-verbal familiar sounds such as a telephone ringing, of tactile stimuli, tastes and smells. Thus, patients lose their factual knowledge about the world, much of which is acquired early in life.

Despite the pervasive nature of the semantic loss, the disorder is nevertheless circumscribed in the sense that non-semantic aspects of cognitive functioning remain remarkably well preserved. Patients do not have difficulty in processing the sounds of language and do not make phonological errors in speech. Moreover sentence construction is grammatically correct. Nor do patients have problems in perceiving visual, tactile, gustatory and olfactory stimuli. They are able to distinguish whether two sensory stimuli are alike and therefore perform well on perceptual matching tasks. The problem lies at the level of assigning identity (meaning) to a stimulus that is apparently perceived normally. Thus, patients are able to repeat words that they do not understand and can reproduce drawings of objects that they cannot recognize. Patients' day-to-day memory also remains relatively well preserved, so they remember appointments and daily events, such as the visit from a friend, can keep track of time and can negotiate their environment without becoming lost. Their preserved day-to-day memory undoubtedly contributes to patients' capacity to retain a high degree of functional independence well into the course of the disease despite severe semantic loss. An additional contributory factor is the fact that patients typically remain physically well and show few neurological signs until late in the disease. When physical signs emerge in advanced disease, these are usually limited to mild Parkinsonian features of akinesia and rigidity.

The course of the disease is one of insidious progression, with gradual increase in severity of semantic impairment. Patients' repertoire of vocabulary becomes increasingly restricted, so that eventually only a few stereotyped phrases remain. At no time, however, is speech output effortful or non-fluent. Patients fail increasingly to recognize the visual environment and may no longer know the function of common objects. Inappropriate behaviours may arise as an integral part of the disease.

Clinical investigations of patients with degenerative dementia commonly include electroencephalography and structural and functional brain imaging. The electroencephalogram in semantic dementia is usually normal, a feature that helps to distinguish it from more common forms of dementia such as Alzheimer's disease in which typically there is slowing of wave forms. Structural brain imaging reveals cerebral atrophy. Computed tomography is generally insufficiently sensitive to reveal clear anatomical differences in the distribution of atrophy between the two cerebral hemispheres and between the different lobes of the brain. Magnetic resonance (MR) imaging, however, typically demonstrates atrophy predominantly of the anterior temporal lobes, and this may be obviously asymmetric, affecting the left or right temporal lobe preferentially. Functional brain imaging using positron emission tomography (PET) or single photon emission tomography (SPECT) shows abnormal function of the anterior cerebral hemispheres, particularly the temporal regions. Appearances may be bilateral and symmetrical or markedly asymmetric affecting disproportionately the left or right hemisphere. The salient clinical features of semantic dementia are summarized in Table 1.

Individual differences

Semantic dementia is a remarkably uniform disorder in the sense that the characteristics of patients' language, their areas of preserved cognition, and their behavioural foibles and idiosyncrasies are surprisingly predictable from one patient to the next. Nevertheless, patients with semantic dementia are not entirely homogeneous. The most notable difference lies in the emphasis of the semantic impairment on the verbal

Table 1. Semantic dementia: summary of clinical features

Insidious onset and progressive course
Impaired word comprehension and naming
Impaired object and face recognition
Preservation of auditory and visual perception
Preservation of day-to-day memories
Behavioural alterations
Neurological abnormalities absent or minimal
Electroencephalography normal
Structural brain imaging: atrophy, particularly of temporal lobes
Functional brain imaging: temporal lobe dysfunction

or non-verbal domain. In some patients the clinical presentation is specific-ally of problems in word comprehension and naming; they recognize objects for which they no longer understand the name, e.g. they can identify a picture of a chair, while failing to understand the meaning of the word *chair*. Such patients are sometimes described as having a fluent form of progressive aphasia (Basso, Capitani and Laiacona, 1988; Poeck and Luzzatti, 1988; Snowden, Neary, Mann et al., 1992; Tyrrell, Warrington, Frackowiak et al., 1990a). In other patients the initial emphasis of impair-ment lies within the visual domain and patients may present, sometimes selectively, with a problem in recognition of familiar faces. Published case reports of patients with progressive prosopagnosia (Evans, Heggs, Antoun et al., 1995; Tyrrell et al., 1990b) are likely to represent early, circum-scribed presentations of semantic dementia. The verbal–non-verbal differ-ence amongst semantic dementia patients appears to reflect anatomical differences in emphasis of pathology in the left and right hemispheres. Patients with greater verbal semantic impairment show greater left temporal atrophy, whereas those with more non-verbal impairment show more right temporal change. Performance differences for verbal and pic-torial material can be demonstrated on the Pyramids and Palm Trees test (Howard and Patterson, 1992), which comprises matched verbal and non-verbal versions of the task. The semantic disorder rarely remains confined to a single domain and a multi-modal semantic impairment typically emerges over the course of the disease.

Demographic features

The main demographic features of semantic dementia are summarized in Table 2. Semantic dementia most commonly has its onset between the ages of 50 and 65 and affects both men and women (Snowden et al., 1996b). The time course of the illness is variable, the median illness duration being approximately 8 years, ranging from 3 to 15 years. Most cases appear to occur sporadically. A history of dementia is documented in a first degree relative in a minority of patients. In view of the poor clinical recognition of semantic dementia and the retrospective nature of family history data it is, however, often difficult to determine with certainty whether the dementia in affected relatives was indeed of the semantic type. There are no known geographical or socio-economic factors that affect incidence. No incidence or prevalence data are currently available. However, the disorder would appear to be relatively rare. Of referrals to our own specialist dementia clinic in Manchester, patients with prototypical semantic dementia accounted for approximately 10% of cases of focal cortical degeneration (frontotemporal lobe degeneration), which in turn accounted for 20–25% of cases of primary degenerative dementia presenting before the age of 65 years. To provide a more concrete guide: for each patient referred with semantic dementia, 50 patients of comparable age were seen with Alzheimer's disease.

Table 2. Semantic dementia: demographic features

Onset usually 50–65 years
Affects both men and women
Mean duration of illness = 8 years, range 3–15 years
May be familial
Rare disorder compared to Alzheimer's disease
No known geographical or socio-economic factors affecting prevalence

---

Anatomy and histopathology

The degenerative process predominantly affects the anterior part of the temporal neocortex, particularly the inferior and middle temporal gyri (Snowden et al., 1996b). The superior temporal gyrus that includes the traditional language region of Wernicke's area is relatively spared. Relatively spared too are medial temporal structures, including the hippocampus, which are critical for formation of new memories. Aside from the temporal lobe atrophy, there is typically some involvement of frontal cortices, particularly the orbital portions. In contrast, parietal and occipital cortices are relatively well preserved. The temporal lobe atrophy usually involves both hemispheres, although often asymmetrically. The emphasis of involvement of left or right temporal lobe reflects the precise pattern of semantic impairment, and is the source of individual differences between patients.

The histopathological changes seen in the brains of deceased individuals are characterized by loss of large pyramidal nerve cells from affected areas of temporal and frontal cortex and a spongiform (microvacuolar) change due to neuronal fallout. There is also a reactive astrocytosis, typically of mild degree. Ballooned neurones and inclusion bodies, conventionally considered pathological hallmarks of 'Pick's disease', are typically absent. This pattern of histopathological change, in which microvacuolation is the prominent feature and in which the histological features of ballooned cells and inclusions are absent, has been referred to as microvacuolar-type or frontal-lobe-degeneration-type (FLD) histology (Brun, Englund, Gustafson et al., 1994). In a minority of cases, however, Pick-type histology may be observed, with severe astrocytic gliosis and the presence of ballooned neurones and inclusion bodies. The pathological features in semantic dementia are distinct from those of Alzheimer's disease. No deposits of ß/A4 amyloid protein are present in any cortical region, nor are there cells containing neurofibrillary tangles or Lewy-body-type inclusions.

The pathological changes in semantic dementia are identical to those seen in other focal degenerative syndromes affecting the anterior parts of the brain; specifically, the behavioural disorder of frontotemporal dementia (Neary, Snowden, Northen et al., 1988) and the language disorder of slowly progressive non-fluent aphasia (Mesulam, 1982). The difference lies only in the anatomical distribution of that pathological change within the anterior cerebral hemispheres (Snowden et al., 1996b). In the case of semantic dementia the predominant involvement is in the anterior temporal lobes, whereas in frontotemporal dementia, although the temporal poles are affected, the major involvement is the frontal cortices. In progressive non-fluent aphasia, the atrophy is markedly asymmetric, the left hemisphere being more affected than the right and there is extensive involvement of the perisylvian language areas. The pathological link between semantic dementia, frontotemporal dementia, and progressive non-fluent aphasia, is reinforced by the observation that some patients exhibit features that overlap these distinct prototypical syndromes, and characteristics of the different syndromes may be manifest in different members of the same family. Terms such as 'lobar atrophy', 'focal cerebral degenerations', 'Pick-complex' or (frontotemporal lobar degeneration) have been adopted as generic terms to distinguish these associated focal forms of dementia from the more common and pathologically distinct form of dementia of Alzheimer's disease.

Is semantic dementia a new disorder?

The term semantic dementia is relatively new. It was introduced a decade ago (Snowden et al., 1989) to encapsulate the multi-modal loss of semantic knowledge that occurs in the face of relatively preserved non-semantic cognitive skills. It has since been adopted by others (Breedin et al., 1994; Funnell, 1995a; 1996; Graham, Becker and Hodges, 1997; Hodges et al., 1992; 1995; Lauro-Grotto, Piccini and Shallice, 1997). Clinical criteria have been published to aid identification of the disorder (Neary, Snowden, Gustafson et al., 1998). There is no doubt that cases of semantic dementia existed prior to contemporary classification. There have been reports in the literature of patients with circumscribed impairments of semantic memory occurring in association with degenerative brain disease, who would now be recognized as having semantic dementia (Schwartz, Marin and Saffran, 1979, 1980; Warrington, 1975). In the more distant past there are reports in the literature of patients with focal temporal lobe atrophy in whom the predominant feature was a lexico-semantic impairment (Pick, 1892; Rosenfeld, 1909). The neurological term 'transcortical sensory aphasia' has historically been applied to this form of language disorder. It is likely that such cases would now be regarded as having semantic dementia, and also that cases of semantic dementia have always existed but that the disorder's clinical distinctiveness has often failed to be recognized.

Why is semantic dementia poorly recognized?

Semantic dementia is not well recognized by medical professionals. There are likely to be several contributory factors underlying this fact. One reason is that semantic dementia is a rare disorder in comparison with other degenerative conditions. Experience of the disorder and its salient characteristics is likely to be limited. Moreover, a common assumption until recently has been that individuals with a primary degenerative dementia (that is, people who are physically well without cerebrovascular and other systemic disease and who have a progressive degeneration of the cerebral cortex) will inevitably have Alzheimer's disease. Indeed, the most common incorrect diagnosis given to patients with semantic dementia is that of Alzheimer's disease.

Misdiagnosis is to some extent understandable. Patients and their relatives do not complain specifically of semantic problems, and may not perceive a difficulty in word comprehension and naming in terms of a problem in language. Rather, they often attribute their progressive semantic disorder to failing memory and will complain that they 'cannot remember anything'. Careful history-taking will reveal that the problem is not one of amnesia in the traditional sense. Patients are able to remember day-to-day events, keep track of time, remember appointments, find their way around without becoming lost, and retain a degree of functional independence that would be incompatible with a classical amnesia. The problem lies in the realm of semantic memory: in knowing what words mean, who people are and what objects are for. Patients may, for example, no longer recognize fruits and vegetables in the supermarket. Nevertheless, the symptoms, taken at face value, may be misinterpreted as indicating amnesia, a characteristic presenting feature of Alzheimer's disease.

The faulty diagnosis is often reinforced by patients' poor performance on conventional memory tests. The latter typically involve learning lists of words or recalling faces or line drawings, all of which may have little meaning for the patient. To complicate matters further, the semantic disorder, even in severely affected patients, may not be immediately apparent at clinical interview. Patients' fluent, effortless speech output gives a superficial impression of a facility with language, which belies the underlying semantic impairment. Moreover, patients may retain conversational vocabulary pertaining to their daily lives, obscuring the magnitude of their anomia. Similarly, patients' preserved ability to negotiate their visual environment and their dexterous manipulation of objects may obscure failures of object recognition. It is only on direct testing of word comprehension and naming, and of face and object recognition, that the disorder becomes evident.

An additional factor hindering recognition is the fact that semantic knowledge does not break down in an all-or-none fashion. Conceptual loss may be partial rather than absolute. A patient may, for example, know that a dog is an animal rather than something to eat, but not know how it differs from a cat. In consequence, patients' use of vocabulary and behaviour with respect to objects in the environment is likely to be broadly appropriate until concepts are very severely degraded relatively late in the disease course. It is perhaps for this reason that patients frequently already have very severe semantic deficits, demonstrable on formal testing, by the time of their initial presentation to medical attention: subtle semantic impairments remain undetected in daily life and do not raise cause for concern.

The foregoing emphasizes the fact that semantic dementia is not easily diagnosed by clinical history alone. Furthermore, since patients remain physically well, there are also no neurological markers that clearly differentiate semantic dementia from the more common dementia of Alzheimer's disease. The semantic impairment, which may be scarcely apparent at clinical interview, becomes strikingly evident on formal testing of naming and word comprehension. Indeed, it is the systematic assessment of patients' language and other cognitive skills that is critical in eliciting patients' semantic disorder and in characterizing the nature of patients' condition. Hence, speech and language therapists and psychologists play a crucial role in identification of the disorder.

Language and its assessment

The salient characteristics of patients' language disorder are summarized in Table 3.

Table 3. Language breakdown in semantic dementia

Spontaneous speech	• Fluent, effortless, often garrulous • Content empty, reliance on generic terms • stereotyped words and phrases • Semantic paraphasias • Preserved phonology and syntax
Comprehension	• Impaired word comprehension • Good syntactic comprehension
Naming	• Profound anomia, semantic errors • No benefit from semantic or phonemic cues
Repetition	• Relatively preserved
Reading	• Fluent reading aloud • Regularization errors (surface dyslexia) • Impaired reading comprehension
Writing	• Fluent execution • Poor spelling to dictation of words with irregular spelling-to-sound correspondence (surface dysgraphia)

Spontaneous speech

Patients speak fluently and effortlessly, with normal articulation and prosody. They may appear garrulous. Utterances are grammatically correct and free from phonological errors. Because of these features, output may give a superficial impression of being normal and it is undoubtedly for this reason that the disorder may not be construed as one of language. More critical examination will, however, typically reveal an emptiness of content, with a reduction in the number of content words, and a tendency on the part of the patient to rely on broad generic terms and stock words and phrases. The repertoire of conversational topics on which patients embark is limited and invariably relates to issues pertaining to their own life. Patients may revert constantly to a single theme. Successive meetings with the patient will highlight the repetitive and stereotyped quality of stock words and phrases and thematic content.

Over-inclusive use of terms such as use of the word *water* to refer to all forms of liquid and frank within-category semantic errors such as saying *sock* for *glove* provide the most obvious clue to the underlying semantic impairment although these may occur relatively infrequently in patients' spontaneous output. The semantic impairment that may be scarcely apparent in general conversation becomes strikingly evident on formal testing of word comprehension and naming.

Comprehension

There is significant loss of understanding of nominal terms. Word comprehension problems can be elicited by a range of standard word definition and word–picture matching tests (e.g. PALPA: Kay, Lesser and Coltheart, 1992) and semantic association tasks (e.g. the Pyramids and Palm Trees test: Howard and Patterson, 1992). A characteristic response when asked the meaning of a word X is: 'What's X? I don't know what that is. I've never heard of X.' Patients emphatically deny all knowledge of the word. Patients typically show a high degree of consistency of performance from one testing session to another. Words that are not understood on one occasion will not be understood on another. This consistency reflects the fact that there is a loss of semantic representation and not merely faulty access to lexical representations.

There is typically a word frequency effect, with common words being better understood than low frequency words. Loss of word meaning does not, however, occur in an all or none fashion, and patients may retain partial information about a word that allows them to make broad categorical judgements while showing impaired knowledge of specific properties or attributes. For example, the word *tiger* may be recognized as the name of an animal, but not understood as referring to the particular animal that is striped, dangerous and is not native to Britain. A tiger may be distinguished conceptually from a tomato or a comb, but not from a cat or a dog. Similarly, a lemon may be understood as 'something to eat' but the patient may have no knowledge of how a lemon differs from an orange or apple. Assessment of word comprehension needs therefore to evaluate knowledge of properties of objects as well as the broad categories into which they fall.

Some patients with semantic dementia appear to show disproportionate degrees of impairment for certain types or categories of information. They have particular difficulty understanding the names of animals and foods and better comprehension of inanimate object names (Basso et al., 1988; Breedin et al., 1994; Snowden et al., 1996b). This phenomenon of 'category specificity' has been observed also in patients with temporal lobe damage resulting from herpes simplex encephalitis (Sartori and Job,

1988; Silveri and Gainotti, 1988; Warrington and Shallice, 1984). A prominent view (Warrington and Shallice, 1984) has been that category differences reflect differences in the types of attributes that make up a concept. Conceptual differentiation between two animals, such as a tiger and lion, is strongly dependent upon their visual appearance. Two fruits, such as an orange and lemon, are distinguished by their shape, colour, smell and taste. That is, sensory properties are critically important. Conversely, inanimate objects, such as a glass and vase are defined conceptually more by their function than by their physical appearance: a glass and vase may have very similar appearance but very different functions. If semantic breakdown were to affect specifically knowledge about sensory properties then this would lead to more severe comprehension impairment for animal and food terms than inanimate object terms. It should be emphasized that this interpretation has not received universal acceptance and the basis for the phenomenon is a continuing subject for debate (e.g. Funnell and Sheridan, 1992; Funnell and De Mornay Davies, 1996). Nevertheless, disproportionate impairment for animal and food concepts appears invariably to be associated with damage to the temporal neocortex as in semantic dementia. In contrast, the converse finding of greater impairment for inanimate object concepts (Warrington and McCarthy, 1983, 1987; Sacchett and Humphreys, 1992) has been associated with lesions outside the temporal neocortex. The anatomical consistency of such findings suggests that category differences cannot solely be attributable to differences in item difficulty. That comprehension impairment might be disproportionately affected for certain concept types has led to the publication of tests that specifically address the issue of category differences in comprehension (McKenna, 1998).

Category dissociations are not apparent in all patients with semantic dementia. However, a class of information that appears commonly to be relatively preserved late into the disease is that relating to number concepts (Diesfeldt, 1993; Snowden et al., 1996b). Patients have no difficulty appreciating the significance of spoken and written numerals, they are able to count money and reckon change. They retain knowledge of arithmetical procedures and may even continue to pursue occupations in accountancy, despite major difficulties in word comprehension and naming. With progression of disease, however, number concepts eventually become impaired.

Language comprehension problems arise principally at the single word level. Comprehension of the syntactic rules of language is typically relatively well preserved. Thus, a patient may respond with ease to the question, 'If the tiger is killed by the lion which animal is dead?' while failing the apparently simpler question, 'Is a tiger bigger than a mouse?'

The former depends on understanding of grammatical relationships, whereas the latter depends on understanding of the lexical terms *tiger* and *mouse*. Standard tests of comprehension of grammar, such as the revised Token test (De Renzi and Faglioni, 1978), and the Test of Reception of Grammar (TROG: Bishop, 1989) are typically performed well. Performance may be compromised to some extent by failure to understand individual lexical items, such as the terms *square* and *circle* in the Token test, yet if demands on lexical understanding are minimized, by the use of commands such as, 'Put this one under that one,' then performance is commonly error free.

Naming

Naming performance is invariably profoundly impaired, whether naming pictures, as in the Boston Naming test (Kaplan, Goodglass, Weintraub et al., 1983) and Graded Naming test (McKenna and Warrington, 1983), or naming from verbal description. Although omission errors (i.e. 'don't know' responses) and superordinate category substitutions (e.g. 'animal' for lion) occur, it is the presence of within-category errors (e.g. 'dog' for lion or elephant) that is characteristic of the condition, and exemplifies the semantic impairment. Another key feature that helps to distinguish the semantic impairment from one of lexical retrieval is the lack of significant benefit to the patient of provision of phonemic prompts (e.g. 'It begins with "l".') or semantically related multiple-choice alternatives (e.g. 'Is it a lion, a tiger or a leopard?'). The reason is that the problem is not one of accessing vocabulary that is potentially available: there is a central loss of the vocabulary itself. Nevertheless, provision of unrelated alternatives (e.g. 'Is it a lion, a lemon or a lamp?') may, in some instances, benefit the patient in yielding the correct response, since partial information may be available sufficient to allow the patient to eliminate incorrect alternatives. Phonemic paraphasic errors in naming are absent. Responses are produced at a normal rate, whether correct or incorrect, and there are never indications of effortful word search or frustrated attempts at word retrieval (tip-of-the-tongue phenomena).

Naming performance is consistent across testing occasions. A failure to name an item on one occasion predicts failure on that same item on successive occasions. There is typically also a close association between word comprehension and naming. The name of an object which is not understood will not normally be produced in a naming task. Category differences that emerge on comprehension tests are also likely to be demonstrated on naming tests.

An additional factor that appears relevant in influencing what vocabulary is retained is its relevance to patients' daily life. It has been demonstrated that vocabulary pertaining to patients' contemporary autobiographical experience is better preserved than non-personally relevant vocabulary (Snowden et al., 1994, 1995). Arguments have been put forward emphasizing the role of patients' preserved day-to-day memory in supporting this personal vocabulary (Snowden et al., 1994, 1995, 1996a, 1999). Assessment of word comprehension and naming should not be restricted to household objects likely to be relevant to the patient's daily life, but should include names of animals, foods and objects, which although relatively common are unlikely to relate directly to the patient's daily routine.

Repetition

Patients are able to repeat words and phrases that they do not understand and in the later stages of disease may show echolalia: a tendency to repeat verbatim and without comprehension what is said to them. Since repetition of complex material is partially mediated in normal subjects by semantics, repetition skills may be compromised to some extent in the face of profound semantic loss. Nevertheless the dissociation between the ability to repeat and the lack of ability to understand what is being repeated is striking. Digit span is typically normal.

Reading

Comprehension of written material mirrors aural comprehension: there is profound loss of meaning of lexical terms, whereas understanding of syntax is well preserved. Reading aloud is fluent and effortless, contrasting with the profound failure to understand what is read. Pronunciation is largely accurate, with normal word stress, provided that words have regular spelling-to-sound correspondences. However, a pattern of reading errors consistent with a 'surface dyslexia' (Patterson, Marshall and Coltheart, 1985) is commonly observed (Breedin et al., 1994; Funnell, 1996; Hodges et al., 1992; Snowden et al., 1989; 1996b). For irregular words patients typically make phonetic regularization errors, e.g. *pint* is read to rhyme with *mint*; *glove* to rhyme with *rove*. Matched reading lists of 'regular' and 'exception' words (Coltheart, Besner, Jonasson et al., 1979; Glushko, 1979) typically elicit striking discrepancies in reading accuracy for the two lists. Some visual substitution errors may occur in reading (e.g. *lamb* read as *lamp*), particularly with progression of disease.

Writing

Patients' writing skills are compromised by their problem in word meaning, and impairment in the ability to convey information in writing mirrors the disorder of spoken language. However, just as oral repetition is relatively preserved, so too is the patients' ability to write to dictation. Writing is executed fluently and effortlessly, albeit without comprehension. Writing to dictation is not, though, error-free and patients exhibit a picture of 'surface dysgraphia': words with irregular correspondence between spelling and sound are 'regularized' (e.g. *caught* spelt as *cort*) (Hodges et al., 1992; Snowden et al., 1989, 1996b). Similar regularization errors occur in oral spelling.

Communication by gesture and pantomime

Just as the tools of spoken language (syntax and phonology) are preserved, so too are patients' motor skills. Nevertheless, patients' ability to communicate by gesture or pantomime is limited by their semantic disorder: by loss of meaning for the information to be conveyed. Patients who are unable to define the meaning of a word orally will not be able to do so by gesture. On the other hand, prior to the onset of visual recognition difficulties, patients may demonstrate the function of an object, which they cannot name, reflecting the dissociation between meaning for visual material and for its linguistic label.

Non-verbal cognition and its assessment

Object and face recognition

Language specialists whose specified role is to assess and treat language problems frequently need to confront the issue of patients' additional cognitive deficits. To what extent do problems outside the language domain contribute to or exacerbate patients' level of functional disability, and to what extent might they compromise the efficacy of therapeutic interventions? The issue is particularly pertinent with respect to patients with semantic dementia. The semantic disorder is not confined to the meaning of words. A patient who does not understand the word *apple* may also fail to recognize a picture of an apple, or indeed a real apple. The patient has a central loss of the concept of 'apple'. Pictorial material that provides a valuable therapeutic aid for many aphasic patients may be of little help in semantic dementia. Assessment needs to determine the extent to which object and picture recognition is compromised. The Pyramids and Palm Trees test (Howard and Patterson, 1992) is useful because it employs the same stimuli in separate written and pictorial versions. Other ways of assessing visual semantic knowledge include picture and object sorting tasks. The patient may, for example, be asked to group pictures of animals according to a particular property, such as whether they are wild or tame, are native to this country or not. Recognition failure, like that for words, is not all or none. Patients may, for example, be able to sort objects into those which are edible and which are non-edible, but be unable to distinguish foods that are normally cooked (e.g. potatoes) and those normally eaten uncooked (e.g. lettuce). Patients may recognize a picture of a camel as depicting an animal, but have no idea how it differs from a dog. They may also recognize and use entirely appropriately their own belongings while failing to recognize other examples of those same objects or pictures of those objects (Snowden et al., 1994).

Problems in recognizing familiar faces occur early in the course of disease. Difficulties are most profound for impersonal faces, such as those of current and past celebrities, and least marked for family and friends with whom the patient maintains daily contact.

In semantic dementia the problem in face and object recognition lies at a semantic level and not at a more elementary level of perceptual processing. Assessment of patients needs not only to determine whether a problem in face or object recognition exists but also to differentiate a semantic basis for that problem from non-semantic perceptual impairment. If the disorder lies at a semantic level, then patients should perform well on perceptual discrimination and matching tests, which require them to say whether two visual stimuli are the same or different or which of a set of stimuli are visually identical. They ought also to be able to copy line drawings normally, despite being unable to draw from memory. Copying a picture of a duck, for example, does not require recognition of identity, whereas drawing a duck from memory depends on knowledge about a duck and its visual appearance. The difference between preserved copying ability and impaired drawing from memory mirrors the dissociation in the verbal domain between relatively good repetition and poor naming. A published test battery that explicitly addresses the different levels at which object recognition problem may arise, and allows discrimination between semantic and non-semantic impairments, is the Birmingham Object Recognition Battery (BORB: Riddoch and Humphreys, 1993). With regard to faces, the prediction in patients with semantic dementia is that patients ought to perform poorly on tests of famous face identity, but relatively well on face matching tasks such as the Facial Recognition Test (Benton, Van Allen, Hamsher et al., 1975; Benton, Hamsher, Varney et al., 1983).

Touch, taste, smell and hearing

The disorder of meaning compromises all sensory modalities. Patients may have difficulty recognizing the identity of textures, tastes, smells, and non-verbal sounds such as the ringing of a telephone or doorbell. Nevertheless, just as the auditory and visual perceptual skills are preserved, so too are patients' primary sensory abilities. Patients have no difficulty detecting the presence of tactile, gustatory, olfactory and auditory stimuli and discriminating whether two stimuli are the same or different.

Spatial skills

Spatial and navigational skills are generally excellent. Patients are able to find their way without becoming lost and may use spatial cues to compensate for object recognition difficulties (for example, by recalling the spatial location of food items on a supermarket shelf). On neuropsychological testing, patients perform well on traditional spatial tests such as line orientation (Benton, Varney and Hamsher, 1978), dot counting, position discrimination, and cube estimation (Warrington and James, 1991). The preservation of spatial skills is an important feature in distinguishing semantic dementia from Alzheimer's disease, since in the latter condition spatial skills are commonly disrupted. It is worth recognizing, however, that performance on putative spatial tasks may be compromised secondarily in semantic dementia patients by failures of perceptual recognition. A patient who, for example, fails to 'locate' their comb or toothbrush, may do so because of impaired recognition of object identity and not because of a problem in spatial localization per se. Evidence that spatial skills are indeed well preserved throughout the course of disease is suggested by qualitative characteristics of patients' behaviour. Patients with semantic dementia, even in advanced disease, (Snowden et al., 1996b) negotiate their environment skilfully, and localize, manipulate and align objects perfectly.

Memory

A feature that is striking on clinical grounds and which helps to distinguish semantic dementia from Alzheimer's disease, along with other features (Table 4), is the apparent preservation of patients' current autobiographical memory. Patients remember appointments and personally relevant events and keep track of time. They have no difficulty remembering on which day to visit the hairdresser, collect the pension, or pay the milkman. They initiate activities of daily living unprompted at the correct time of day and do not lose track of tasks in which they are engaged. They negotiate the environment without becoming lost. If they move home they have no difficulty learning their new surroundings. In contrast, they show a gross breakdown in impersonal, factual (semantic) knowledge about the world, including knowledge about public figures and important world events.

Table 4. Main clinical differences between semantic dementia and Alzheimer's disease

	Semantic dementia	Alzheimer's disease
Language	• Selective semantic disorder. • Fluent, effortless, no word search. • Maintains line of thought. Stereotyped phrases. • Semantic paraphasias.	• No selective semantic disorder. • Hesitant, word retrieval difficulties. • Loses line of thought. Incomplete. • Incomplete sentences. • Verbal and phonemic errors.
Perception	• Impaired object identity. • Good perceptual skills.	• Impaired perceptual skills.
Calculation	• Preserved early in course.	• Impaired early in course.
Spatial orientation	• Preserved.	• Impaired early in course.
Memory	• Day-to-day memory preserved.	• Day-to-day memory impaired.

In our own studies we have demonstrated preserved object-specific spatial location memory in patients with semantic dementia. Nevertheless, the preservation of autobiographical memory is not easily captured by standard memory tests since these typically involve lists of words, faces or line drawings that may have little meaning for the patient. Evaluation of the status of patients' memory needs to include questions regarding personal orientation and autobiographically relevant events, supported by ecological observation of patients in their daily lives.

Motor skills

Motor actions are carried out dexterously and effortlessly. Activities with high motor executive demands, such as painting, sewing or playing golf, may continue to be pursued with a high level of proficiency, a feature that is important in distinguishing semantic dementia from Alzheimer's disease. Practical skills are, however, compromised to some degree by patients' semantic loss: for example, a difficulty in cooking arises because patients no longer recognize individual ingredients or do not understand the words of a recipe.

Behavioural changes

Although the semantic deficits are the salient and defining characteristic of the disorder, a number of behavioural changes have been described

(Snowden et al., 1996b). Recognition of these behaviours is important because they may represent the most problematic aspect of the condition from the point of view of patient management and the greatest source of burden to carers. They may also complicate therapeutic interventions.

Patients are commonly described as self-centred and lacking in their former sympathy and empathy for others. They may be inflexible and intransigent and have difficulty seeing others' point of view. They may appear mean and lacking in their former generosity. They commonly have a preference for routine and will clock-watch and carry out activities at precisely the same time each day. They may develop meaningless rituals or compulsions. Their behavioural repertoire becomes narrowed and they frequently become preoccupied with one or two activities, such as doing jigsaws, and they pursue these relentlessly to the detriment of domestic and occupational responsibilities. Moreover, they may become mentally preoccupied by one or two themes that they repeat incessantly. Although such themes may include their own 'memory' problems, patients frequently rationalize their semantic difficulties with trivial explanations such as: 'I'm out of practice.' Patients may show hypersensitivity to sensory stimuli and overreact to light touch or to ostensibly innocuous environmental sounds such as birdsong. They may be oblivious to danger, a feature that is probably linked to their loss of conceptual knowledge about the world. Patients commonly show narrowed food preferences and usually favour sweet foods. The behavioural changes in semantic dementia have a compulsive quality, although the affective responses of anxiety and release from anxiety associated with frank obsessional-compulsive disorder are absent.

Management

Patients with semantic dementia need to be accurately identified and distinguished from patients with Alzheimer's disease. From a purely medical point of view, differentiation is important because of different implications for pharmacological treatment. Over recent years a number of new therapies have been introduced for Alzheimer's disease, based upon the known abnormalities in the cholinergic system in Alzheimer patients. Neurochemical studies of semantic dementia patients, although limited, have failed to indicate a comparable cholinergic abnormality. Cholinergic-based medications devised for Alzheimer's disease are therefore inappropriate. From a wider perspective, differentiation is important because semantic dementia has unique implications for management and in particular the types of interventions considered by speech and language therapists.

Patients with semantic dementia have impaired abstract knowledge about the world and this includes verbal as well as non-verbal concepts. Our own studies have suggested that concepts (words, objects, etc.) relevant to the patient's daily life are better retained than those that have no personal relevance (Snowden et al., 1994,1995,1996a, 1999). Names of personal acquaintances were shown to be better retained than celebrity names. Names of places relevant to the patient's own life were understood better than non-personally relevant place names. Thus, the word *postman* may be understood better than the word *milkman* if the patient has personal daily experience of the postman delivering letters to the home, but purchases milk from the supermarket.

We have demonstrated that the role of personal experience extends also to object recognition (Snowden et al., 1994). Objects belonging to a patient, such as her own comb and kettle, were recognized better than alternative examples of those same objects. Moreover, there was a significant effect of topographical context. Objects were recognized better in their usual location in the patient's home (e.g. a kettle on the worktop in the kitchen) than when they were placed in an incongruous location (e.g. a kettle in the bath). We have argued that the beneficial effect of autobiographical relevance results from patients' preserved autobiographical memory: concepts which would otherwise be lost in their abstract sense have some meaning to the patient if they are framed within the context of the patient's ongoing daily experience.

Experience may also determine the precise nature of information that the patient has available. It has previously been indicated that patients may not have normal conceptual understanding of words, even when those words are used entirely appropriately in conversation. Concept knowledge may be partial. We have demonstrated (Snowden et al., 1995) that patients' understanding may be limited to that aspect of meaning that is pertinent to the patients' daily life. Thus, a patient understood the word *oil* to refer to the substance used for her central heating, but her understanding did not extend beyond that limited personal domain. A similar feature is observed with regard to object recognition. A patient of ours recognized a peg as the object used to close cereal packets (in accordance with her own personal use of pegs), but had no knowledge of its usual function. Another recognized a vase as the object for holding pencils (consistent with its use in the patient's home), but had no knowledge of its other possible functions.

There are evident implications of these autobiographical effects for patient management. Of particular importance is that speech and language therapy input is more likely to be beneficial if this takes place in patients' own surroundings using as referents patients' own belongings, than in the abstract setting of a clinical consulting room using standard pictorial materials. Patients who recognize their own but not other examples of the same object evidently have difficulty generalizing across exemplars. Training using a set of pictures would be unlikely to show transfer to patients' daily life. Moreover, the autobiographical context of a patient's own surroundings acts as a meaningful reference with respect to which concepts can be applied. There is another clear implication. If patients' daily experience is important in supporting residual concept knowledge then the nature of that experience must also be important. Patients with a rich and varied lifestyle who pursue a variety of activities have a wider scope for maintenance of conceptual knowledge about the world than patients with a restricted lifestyle. Thus, there are rational, theoretical grounds for helping patients to maintain activities and social interactions. The regular and direct involvement of patients in activities within the framework of a daily routine is vital.

Patients' ability to pursue activities independently is inevitably compromised by their semantic loss: both by problems in verbal communication and by failure of face and object recognition. Semantic impairment can lead to serious consequences. For example, a patient who had difficulty recognizing objects placed bleach into the bath instead of bubble bath. Another placed her hand into boiling oil because of her lack of knowledge of its potential danger. Nevertheless, aspects of preserved ability can be exploited to reduce the consequences of patients' deficits. That topographical context confers an advantage for object recognition means that objects should always be stored in the same place. To prevent a patient mistaking bleach for bubble bath, the two should be stored separately, only the latter being left in the vicinity of the bath. That patients are able to match for visual similarity and can remember spatial locations means that they can shop for food items, even when they have severe object recognition difficulties. A patient of ours spontaneously adopted a strategy of taking empty containers and food packets with her when shopping. She could recall the general location of the items that she was in the habit of buying and would then match up the empty packets with goods on the supermarket shelves in order to select the correct purchase. Replacing household items, including food products, with identical items helps the patient, since the patient can recognize visual similarity but may not understand conceptual similarity between visually dissimilar items. Brand loyalty needs to be observed!

Understanding patients' semantic problems is a prerequisite for understanding patients' behaviour. Some behavioural changes may arise as a direct consequence of the patient's semantic disorder. One patient's wife became distressed when her husband began to urinate in the waste-paper bin. Initially interpreted as 'anti-social' behaviour the problem was found to arise as a result of his difficulties in object recognition: he no longer understood the different functions of the waste bin and the toilet. Another patient failed to open the front door when the hospital transport arrived to take him to day care. This was initially interpreted as lack of compliance and a refusal to attend. However, it transpired that the patient did not recognize the significance of the doorbell ringing and the knocking at the door, and therefore quite naturally did not respond. The problem was overcome by establishing new arrangements for his collection.

The foregoing emphasizes the importance of understanding patients, in their areas both of strength and of deficit. The former, such as patients' preserved visuospatial skills, provide the basis for compensatory strategies. The latter will guide management. To what extent, however, might it also be possible to re-train lost concepts?

There is a large body of anecdotal evidence that suggests that in semantic dementia some new learning is possible and this new learning may include what is traditionally construed as semantic knowledge as well as event memory. In our own experience, patients have effectively learnt the names of new acquaintances and the names of medicines prescribed to them. A patient who sold her home learnt the name of the buyers involved in the house sale and she used the name appropriately in conversation. Patients who moved home had no difficulty learning their new environment and could find their way without becoming lost. Even a patient with very severe semantic dementia who moved into a residential home learnt without difficulty her way around the multi-storey building and annexe. Other patients have learnt without difficulty the days on which they attend a day-centre, even though day-care attendance has been organized late in the course of the patient's illness. A patient who failed to recognize a toaster when her husband first purchased it quickly learnt its function and could provide an elaborate and impressive demonstration of its use.

Such evidence of new learning is complemented by findings reported by Swales and Johnson (1992). These authors demonstrated that a patient with semantic breakdown resulting from herpes simplex encephalitis was able to relearn lost semantic concepts.

These observations at first sight suggest optimism in the potential efficacy of concept retraining. A note of caution is, however, warranted. First, as already alluded to, if patients' knowledge is affected by experiential relevance, then retraining word or object meaning in an abstract sense is unlikely to be beneficial. Words and objects need to be linked to a meaningful autobiographical context. To take a concrete example: a patient who was in the habit of preparing a gin and tonic for her husband in the evening ceased to place a slice of lemon in his drink despite the availability of lemons in the kitchen. Assessment revealed that she no longer recognized lemons. Attempts to teach her the general concept of lemons and their range of possible functions were futile and had no effect on her method of gin and tonic preparation. A strategy with more practical benefit would be to re-teach the very specific activity of preparing a gin and tonic, involving the slicing and inclusion of a slice of lemon!

Second, new and reacquired concepts are maintained only so long as they are pertinent to patients' daily life and are continually rehearsed and refreshed. A patient who no longer recognized a boiled egg was effectively retaught what it was and how to eat it and did so appropriately and unprompted on subsequent mornings. However, if several days elapsed without him being given a boiled egg at breakfast time, his knowledge was lost and he had to be retaught. A similar feature is observed with vocabulary learning. Our patient, who had no difficulty learning the names of the prospective purchasers of her home and used those names spontaneously in conversation, denied all familiarity with those names when they were presented to her some months after completion of the house sale. Funnell (1995b) has reported comparable findings. Although reteaching concepts of vegetables showed some initial benefit, following an interval without practice all gains were lost. In summary, the available evidence suggests that patients are able to learn, and indeed may succeed in relearning some lost vocabulary. However, such reacquired knowledge is tenuous and can be maintained only so long as it forms an integral part of the patient's daily life.

Conclusion

Semantic dementia is a distinct cerebral disorder that requires detailed and systematic analysis of language and non-verbal cognitive skills for its accurate identification. Speech and language therapists and psychologists have a crucial role. Effective management of patients with semantic dementia requires a clear understanding of patients' underlying disorder and promotion of understanding in others. It also requires recognition of patients' preserved cognitive skills so that appropriate compensatory strategies can be developed. Involvement of patients in a range of activities helps to support and maintain existing concepts and patients' functional independence. Retraining of some concepts may be possible. However, broad, abstract training of concepts is unlikely to be successful and indeed any reacquired knowledge would be unlikely to show transference to patients' daily life. Retraining should focus on specific, personally relevant items for which restoration would confer a practical benefit in daily life.

Patients with semantic dementia exhibit unique patterns of cognitive and behavioural symptomatology which demand novel approaches to treatment and management. It is in this endeavour that speech and language therapists and psychologists have a challenging and pivotal role.

References

Basso A, Capitani E, Laiacona M (1988) Progressive language impairment without dementia: a case with isolated category specific semantic defect. Journal of Neurology, Neurosurgery and Psychiatry 51: 1201–07.

Benton AL, Van Allen MW, Hamsher K de S, Levin HS, (1975) Test of facial recognition. Iowa: University of Iowa Hospitals.

Benton AL, Varney NR, Hamsher K de S (1978) Visuo-spatial judgement: a clinical test. Archives of Neurology 35: 364–67.

Benton AL, Hamsher K de S, Varney NR, Spreen O (1983) Contributions to Neuropsychological Assessment: A Clinical Manual. Oxford: Oxford University Press.

Bishop D (1989) TROG Test of Reception of Grammar. Abingdon: Thomas Leach.

Breedin SD, Saffran EM, Coslett HB (1994) Reversal of the concreteness effect in a patient with semantic dementia. Cognitive Neuropsychology 11: 617–60.

Brun A, Englund B, Gustafson L, Passant U, Mann DMA, Neary D, Snowden JS (1994) Consensus Statement. Clinical and neuropathological criteria for frontotemporal dementia. Journal of Neurology, Neurosurgery and Psychiatry 4: 416–18.

Coltheart M, Besner D, Jonasson JT, Davelaar E (1979) Phonological encoding in a lexical decision task. Quarterly Journal of Experimental Psychology 31: 489–507.

De Renzi E, Faglioni P (1978) Normative data and screening power of a shortened version of the token test. Cortex 14: 41–49.

Diesfeldt HFA (1993) Progressive decline of semantic memory with preservation of number processing and calculation. Behavioural Neurology 6: 239–42.

Evans JJ, Heggs AJ, Antoun N, Hodges JR (1995) Progressive prosopagnosia associated with selective right temporal lobe atrophy: a new syndrome? Brain 118: 1–13.

Funnell E (1995a) Objects and properties: a study of the breakdown of semantic memory. Memory 3: 497–518.

Funnell E (1995b) Semantic dementia. Conference proceedings – Assessment of Dementia, July 1995: University of London.

Funnell E (1996) Response biases in oral reading: an account of the co-occurrence of surface dyslexia and semantic dementia. Quarterly Journal of Experimental Psychology 49A: 417–46.

Funnell E, De Mornay Davies P (1996) JBR: a reassessment of concept familiarity and a category-specific disorder for living things. Neurocase 2: 461–74.

Funnell E, Sheridan J (1992) Categories of knowledge? Unfamiliar aspects of living and non-living things. Cognitive Neuropsychology 9: 135–53.

Glushko RJ (1979) The organisation and activation of orthographic knowledge in reading aloud. Journal of Experimental Psychology: Human Perception and Performance 5: 674–91.

Graham KS, Becker JT, Hodges JR (1997) On the relationship between knowledge and memory for pictures: evidence from the study of patients with semantic dementia and Alzheimer's disease. Journal of the International Neuropsychological Society 3: 534–44.

Hodges JR, Patterson K, Oxbury S, Funnell E (1992) Semantic dementia: progressive fluent aphasia with temporal lobe atrophy. Brain 115: 1783–1806.

Hodges JR, Graham N, Patterson K (1995) Charting the progression of semantic dementia: implications for the organization of semantic memory. Memory 3: 463–95.

Howard D, Patterson K (1992) The Pyramids and Palm Trees Test. Bury St Edmunds: Thames Valley Test Company..

Kaplan E, Goodglass H, Weintraub S, Segal H (1983) Boston Naming Test. Philadelphia: Lea and Febiger.

Kay J, Lesser R, Coltheart M (1992) Psycholinguistic Assessments of Language Processing in Aphasia (PALPA). Hove: Lawrence Erlbaum Associates.

Lauro-Grotto R, Piccini C, Shallice T (1997) Modality-specific operations in semantic dementia. Cortex 33: 593–622.

McKenna P (1998) The Category Specific Names Test. Hove: Lawrence Erlbaum Associates.

McKenna P, Warrington EK (1983) Graded Naming Test. Windsor: NFER-Nelson.

Mesulam MM (1982) Slowly progressive aphasia without generalised dementia. Annals of Neurology 11: 592–98.

Neary D, Snowden JS, Gustafson L, Passant U, Stuss D, Black S, Freedman M, Kertesz A, Robert PH, Albert M, Boone K, Miller B, Cummings J, Benson DF (1998) Frontotemporal lobar degeneration. A consensus on clinical diagnostic criteria. Neurology 51: 1546–54.

Neary D, Snowden JS, Northen B, Goulding PJ (1988) Dementia of frontal lobe type. Journal of Neurology, Neurosurgery and Psychiatry 51: 353–61.

Patterson KE, Marshall JC, Coltheart M (1985) Surface Dyslexia: Neuropsychological and Cognitive Studies of Phonological Reading. Hove and London: Erlbaum.

Pick A (1892) Über die Beziehungen der senilen Hirnatrophie zur Aphasie. Prager Medizinische Wochenschrift 17: 165–67.

Poeck K, Luzzatti C (1988) Slowly progressive aphasia in three patients. The problem of accompanying neuropsychological deficit. Brain 111: 151–68.

Riddoch J, Humphreys GW (1993) BORB: Birmingham Object Recognition Battery. Hove: Lawrence Erlbaum Associates.

Rosenfeld M (1909) Die partielle Grosshirnatrophie. Zeitschrift fur Psychologie und Neurologie 14: 115–30.

Sacchett C, Humphreys GW (1992) Calling a squirrel a squirrel but a canoe a wigwam: a category specific deficit for artefactual object and body parts. Cognitive Neuropsychology 9: 73–86.

Sartori G, Job R (1988) The oyster with four legs: a neuropsychological study on the interaction of vision and semantic information. Cognitive Neuropsychology 5: 105–32.

Schwartz MF, Marin OSM, Saffran EM (1979) Dissociations of language function in dementia: a case study. Brain and Language 7: 277–306.

Schwartz MF, Saffran EM, Marin OSM (1980) Fractionating the reading process in dementia: evidence for word-specific print-to-sound associations. In Coltheart M, Patterson K, Marshall JC, (Eds) Deep Dyslexia. London: Routledge Paul.

Silveri MC, Gainotti G (1988) Interaction between vision and language in category-specific impairment. Cognitive Neuropsychology 5: 677–709.

Snowden JS, Goulding PJ, Neary D (1989) Semantic dementia: a form of circumscribed atrophy. Behavioural Neurology 2: 167–82.

Snowden JS, Neary D, Mann DMA, Goulding PJ, Testa HJ (1992) Progressive language disorder due to lobar atrophy. Annals of Neurology 31: 174–83.

Snowden JS, Griffiths H, Neary D (1994) Semantic dementia: autobiographical contribution to preservation of meaning. Cognitive Neuropsychology 11: 265–88.

Snowden JS, Griffiths HL, Neary D (1995) Autobiographical experience and word meaning. Memory 3: 225–46.

Snowden JS, Griffiths HL, Neary D (1996a) Semantic-episodic memory interactions in semantic dementia: implications for retrograde memory function. Cognitive Neuropsychology 13: 1101–37.

Snowden JS, Neary D, Mann DMA (1996b) Frontotemporal Lobar Degeneration: Frontotemporal Dementia, Progressive Aphasia, Semantic Dementia. London: Churchill-Livingstone.

Snowden JS, Griffiths HL, Neary D (in press) The impact of autobiographical experience on meaning: reply to Graham, Lambon Ralph and Hodges. Cognitive Neuropsychology 16

Swales M, Johnson R (1992) Patients with semantic memory loss: can they relearn lost concepts. Neuropsychological Rehabilitation 2: 295–305.

Tyrrell PJ, Warrington EK, Frackowiak RSJ, Rossor MN (1990a) Heterogeneity in progressive aphasia due to focal cortical atrophy. A clinical and PET study. Brain 113: 1321–36.

Tyrrell PJ, Warrington EK, Frackowiak RSJ, Rossor MN (1990b) Progressive degeneration of the right temporal lobe studied with positron emission tomography. Journal of Neurology, Neurosurgery and Psychiatry 53: 1046–50.

Warrington EK (1975) The selective impairment of semantic memory. Quarterly Journal of Experimental Psychology 27: 635–57.

Warrington EK, McCarthy RA (1983) Category-specific access dysphasia. Brain 106: 859-78.

Warrington EK, McCarthy RA (1987) Categories of knowledge: further fractionations and an attempted integration. Brain 110: 1273–96.

Warrington EK, Shallice T (1984) Category specific semantic impairments. Brain 107: 829–54.

Warrington EK, James M (1991) The Visual Object and Space Perception Battery. Bury St Edmonds: Thames Valley Test Company.

CHAPTER 9

Language and knowledge: knowing and thinking in the absence of language

ROSEMARY VARLEY

Introduction

There are case reports of individuals with severe aphasia, resulting in minimal ability to understand spoken language, to read or write, or to produce spoken language beyond the level of stereotypic utterances, but who behave in ways that indicate that they still have an elaborate knowledge base about their world available to them. Such individuals may act appropriately on objects within the environment – electric kettles are filled with water, and not tea-bags, and are plugged into an electricity socket and not placed upon the hob of a cooker or inside a microwave. Some individuals may drive cars and are able to live alone, organizing care needs such as food and personal hygiene. In addition, despite a global impairment of language, these individuals may seek to communicate with others through extraordinarily resourceful use of a range of communicative tools such as gesture, drawing, and conveying different attitudinal states through varied prosodic marking of a stereotypic utterance. These severely aphasic people are apparently still capable of formulating messages and understanding the communicative intentions of others, despite profound difficulty in manipulating language forms in both comprehension and production performances. It is not the case that all severely aphasic people show a dissociation between knowledge of language and knowledge of non-linguistic elements of their world. There are also reports of broader conceptual and cognitive involvement in global aphasia.

In addition to language impairment occurring with and without broader deficits in cognition, there are individuals whose language knowledge is largely retained but who show impaired performances on tasks requiring novel reasoning. This group of patients often have lesions of the prefrontal cortex, and the difficulties they experience are sometimes labelled as 'dysexecutive syndrome'.

These patient groups who demonstrate a dissociation between their abilities in language and non-language cognitive abilities are important groups for exploring the relationships between language and other high-level cognitive abilities such as conceptual knowledge, thought, and reasoning. The issues of language, concepts, and thought are complex ones, and there is little empirical evidence to help in evaluating competing claims of different theorists. Carruthers (1996) provides some useful distinctions to assist in structuring debate about the relation between language and thinking. He identifies three broad approaches to the role of language in other areas of cognition.

1. A *communicative* conception: language is seen as a function dedicated to interpersonal communication – that is, the exchange of ideas and information between two individuals. It is an approach that suggests that natural language is a system which is separate from that of thought and conceptual knowledge. By this view, aphasia would not result in non-language cognitive failures. At first sight, the reports of individuals with severe aphasia, but relatively intact abilities in non-language domains, would appear to provide support for a communicative conception of language.

2. A *cognitive* conception: language is seen as having a central role in human cognition and in thought, in addition to a role in interpersonal exchange. Carruthers, an advocate of a cognitive view, suggests that certain thoughts can be instantiated only in language. By this view, aphasic individuals with certain forms of language impairment would also be impaired in some forms of thought.

3. A *supra-communicative* view: this is a compromise position between the opposing cognitive and communicative views and suggests that to adopt purely a communicative conception of language ignores the introspective evidence that quite a lot of our conscious thinking seems to occur in language or inner speech. Faced with a complex problem to solve, we are often aware that we mentally 'talk through' possible solutions. But, rather than suggesting, as a proponent of a cognitive conception would, that the inner speech constitutes the thought, the compromise supra-communicative view proposes that language supports and scaffolds certain forms of thinking and reasoning (e.g. Clark, 1998; Dennett, 1991).

This chapter is divided into three sections. The first section addresses the relationship between lexical-semantic knowledge (i.e. meaning attached to the words of the linguistic system) and conceptual knowledge (i.e. the hypothesized set of abstract domain-free knowledge); the second, the role of natural language grammar in certain forms of thought; and finally, there will be an evaluation of the evidence from patients with frontal lobe lesions to establish what other cognitive processes might be involved in high-level thinking.

Lexical-semantics and conceptual-semantics

The psycholinguistic processing models, which have exerted a profound influence on research into and management of aphasic disorders over the past two decades, often propose a level of processing which, in comprehension, is post-linguistic and in production, a level that is pre-linguistic (e.g. Butterworth, 1989; Garrett, 1982). In Garrett's model of sentence production, an initial 'message formulation' stage is postulated. This operates at a language-independent conceptual level. An event is conceptualized in terms of the action involved and the entities that are linked together in that action. For example, I observe a child trying to retrieve a ball that is floating on a pond. She tries to knock the ball towards the bank using a long stick. This event involves various entities – the child, the ball, the stick and the pond – and various actions – floating, knocking, retrieving, and their combination – in order to characterize a particular event. This stage is hypothesized as being at a conceptual level and prior to language encoding. Linguistic encoding of the conceptualized event occurs at subsequent 'functional' and 'positional' levels, where lexical-semantic representations for the various entities and actions are activated, phonological forms are retrieved, and the components of the event are assembled into a grammatical structure.

Garrett's model combines well with multi-tiered lexical processing models, such as that of Butterworth (1989). The Butterworth model, and many other models within a psycholinguistic tradition (e.g. Levelt, 1989; Saffran, 1982), are often described as two-stage lexical models. This is because they postulate two separate stages in lexical retrieval: first, a semantic stage involving access to an abstract semantic representation, or *lemma*, and second, a phonological stage involving mapping the semantic representation to an appropriate phonological form, or *lexeme*. Hence a semantic representation encapsulating 'a fleshy plant, found in deserts' would be mapped to the phonological form *cactus*. (See Funnell, Chapter 1, this volume, for a more detailed treatment of these issues.) In reality, however, these two-stage lexical processing models are better described as three-tier models. Two-stage output models include, in addition to semantic and phonological lexicons, a pre-linguistic or conceptual level of processing. This is labelled as the 'semantic system' in Butterworth's formulation, (which is easy to confuse with the postulated second stage – the 'semantic lexicon'). There is, in general, a considerable lack of clarity in both exposition of the distinction between conceptual and semantic systems, and in the terminology that is used to refer to these hypothesized separate tiers.

The evidence to support a separation between a conceptual level and a semantic level often comes from observations of people with aphasia who conform to the description given in the opening paragraph. Despite difficulties in selecting the picture of a toothbrush when presented with the spoken or written word, or in labelling the same picture, an individual can act appropriately upon the object when it is presented to them. The toothbrush will be used to scrub teeth and not as a pen, or a hairbrush, or a tool to stir tea. In attempts to name the picture, the individual may produce a good pantomime of using a toothbrush. All this suggests that knowledge or a concept of a toothbrush is available at some level. These clinical reports of dissociations between knowledge of the object and linguistic-semantic knowledge have been confirmed in case studies of aphasic patients. Howard and Orchard-Lisle (1984), for example, report the case of JCU who was able to make accurate semantic judgements about pictures, despite impairments in lexical-semantic processing. This study used a prototype version of the Pyramids and Palm Trees Test (Howard and Patterson, 1992). In this test, the patient is presented with a stimulus picture (e.g. a pyramid) and then asked to decide which of two response choices (e.g. a fir tree and a palm tree) goes with the pyramid. Investigations using this task have indicated that dissociations between knowledge of word meaning and knowledge of picture meaning are not uncommon (see also Warrington and Shallice, 1984; Bub, Black, Hampson et al.,1988; McCarthy and Warrington, 1988).

There are different ways of accounting for this dissociation. One is to propose the third tier of abstract conceptual representation within a processing model as is included within the Butterworth model. The idea here is that all inputs from different modalities – i.e. tactile, olfactory, auditory-phonological, auditory-non-phonological (e.g. the sound of a dog barking) – would ultimately contact an abstract central (input/output) conceptual representation and the meaning of input would then be derived. But the three-tier architecture raises far more questions than it resolves. In comprehension, why would processing of a word proceed beyond the linguistic-semantic level? What added value would contact with the abstract concept of 'dog' contribute beyond the already accessed lexical-semantic information? Nor is it clear of what the abstract conceptual representation of an item might consist – what is the abstract 'essence of dog'? Butterworth's model neatly avoids some of these difficulties by proposing that the linguistic-semantic system is not a knowledge store, but a transcoding system that, in word-finding, takes in a semantic code from the semantic system and matches it to an appropriate entry in the phonological lexicon. Thus the lexical-semantic system is operating rather as a psycholinguistic match-maker, pairing conceptual information with a matched phonological partner. Such a proposal avoids the redundancy of having lexical-semantic and conceptual-semantic representation but runs into serious issues of biological plausibility. How would such a transcoding mechanism work – how would it 'know' how to match a conceptual code to a phonological one? If the answer to this question is along the lines 'because of the associations that have developed between phonological items and meaning representations,' then why is an extra piece of processing machinery required? If a network of associations is in place, then it is possible to cut out the middleman (the transcoding device) and map directly between meaning and form.

An alternative architecture to account for the dissociation between performances on lexical-semantic and picture-semantic tasks is the proposal that there are modality-specific semantic systems (e.g. Warrington, 1975: see Chapter 1, this book). Rather than an three-tier architecture, there are instead semantic systems operating in parallel and processing different types of input (e.g. words versus objects/pictures). The notion of separate semantic stores is often criticized as a uneconomical explanation of the nature of semantic knowledge as it appears to involve reduplication of information. But the hierarchically organized models may be equally unparsimonious. If a three-tier model postulates independent semantic and conceptual representation, then this represents redundancy in a vertical dimension, while in parallel store models the redundancy operates in a horizontal dimension. The multiple store models perhaps have greater biological plausibility. Within the brain there are separate processing routes for inputs from different sensory modalities: hence it is possible to identify auditory cortex in the temporal lobe, visual cortex in the occipital lobe, and so on. Surrounding the primary sensory cortex are regions of secondary or association cortex where higher-level perceptual processing begins. A percept is an abstract category used in recognizing inputs. For example, pyramids occur in different shapes and sizes. We encounter two- and three-dimensional pyramids; we find tall, thin pyramids and short, squat ones. Although these instances of pyramids differ in basic sensory information, they possess commonalities of form that permit identification as members of the category (or percept) of pyramids. At the level of perceptual processing, there will be local connections between percepts which frequently co-occur. Hence a pyramid visual percept becomes linked to percepts of palm trees, and images of shepherds are linked to sheep, but not to mice. Similar patterns of local connectivity will be found based on associative learning in other processing systems – thus there will be connections within the linguistic system between items such as *new* and *potatoes*.

In addition to local connectivity, there is connectivity between different modalities. The human brain is remarkable for the amount of polymodal association cortex it contains. These are brain areas that allow the mixing of inputs from different processing modalities so that linguistic percepts can be interlinked with picture and object percepts. Hence our integrated sense (or 'concept') of 'dog' may be the result of this polymodal and widely distributed knowledge of dogs. There is some empirical support for this view from disconnection-type disorders. Beauvois (1982) described 'optic aphasia', where patients are unable to name pictures or objects, but are able to name the same item in response to a verbal defin- ition or when the patient is allowed to touch the object, thus permitting linguistic information to be accessed via a tactile route. Visual perception does not appear impaired in such patients as they are able to make categor- ization decisions with pictures and objects. The deficit appears to involve linkage of information across modalities. This type of disorder, together with other forms of 'disconnection' syndrome, suggest a disturbance to the polymodal integrating system and a loss of the links between all elements of a concept.

Both multiple semantic store models and three-tier models are, in terms of the views of the role of language in thinking, compatible with a communicative conception of language in that the lexical-semantic system operates as an autonomous system independent from the conceptual level. Following a lesion, if the conceptual representation (in the three-tier system) or non-linguistic semantic systems (in a multi-store model) are undamaged, there is the possibility of spared conceptual knowledge. But the situation may be more complicated. Not all percepts have an elaborate polymodal representation. For example, abstract words such as 'democ- racy' and 'honesty' may have little representation outside of the linguistic system – most people would be hard pressed to respond to the question 'What does democracy smell like?'. The notion of imageability – defined by Paivio, Yuille and Madigan as 'a word's capacity to arouse non-verbal images' (1968: 11) – is familiar in the assessment of semantic disorders in aphasia. Low imageability, abstract words may be particularly vulnerable to loss in aphasia because of their lack of representation in regions outside of the lesioned language zone. This view is more compatible with supra- communicative and cognitive views in that language support is essential in order to entertain ideas about certain things (like 'democracy' or 'informed consent').

Multiple semantic store and three-tier models allow some account to be given of dissociations between linguistic-semantic knowledge and picture/object knowledge in severe aphasia. In addition, although whole-sale conceptual impairment may not be a component of semantic-level aphasia, in individual cases it may co-occur with aphasia because of the scale and extent of a brain lesion. Lesions which either extend to brain areas mediating other semantic stores, or damage the polymodal areas which 'glue together' a distributed representation, may result in broader conceptual failures. The lesions in global forms of aphasia can be very large (e.g. Kertesz, Lesk and McCabe, 1977) and it is not surprising that, although some dissociations between language and non-language cognition have been reported within this patient group, there are persistent reports of cognitive impairment accompanying these severe aphasia disorders (Kertesz, 1988; van Mourik, Verschaeve, Boon et al., 1992). In this instance, the association between linguistic and conceptual impairment would be a consequence of an accident of geography (or adjacent brain regions) rather than a true functional interrelationship between language and thought.

Lexical-semantic knowledge therefore can be considered to form a component of conceptual knowledge. This is true, in particular, for low imageability, abstract constructs. I have suggested that if lexical-semantic knowledge is disrupted, then other components of the concept – visual-semantic knowledge, for example – may still be available to the individual. This would allow a person to retain a concept despite the loss of linguistic knowledge. The next section will address the issue of grammar in thinking – do our thoughts consist of sentence-like objects, and if so, what are the implications of severe agrammatic aphasia for thinking?

Grammar and thinking

Introspective evidence suggests that when we are given a complex problem to solve, we often use inner speech to reason out a solution. This is not to say that this is the only mode of mental representation that we are able to utilize: we are also able to think in images. But a considerable amount of our conscious thinking appears to take place in inner speech. The introspective evidence has led some philosophers and other behavioural scientists to suggest that certain thoughts can be entertained only in a sentence-like or propositional code. The types of thoughts that are proposed as candidates for propositional thinking are those that have a degree of embedded internal structure. An example may help to clarify the issue here. Reasoning out what another individual might know or be thinking is often referred to as 'theory of mind' – i.e. knowing that other individuals have minds that have different contents to your own mind. A widely used theory of mind task is the 'Smarties' or 'changed container/appearance' test (also known, more technically, as a test of 'first order false belief'). The Smarties task involves presenting a participant with a tube of Smarties, which is opened to reveal that the contents are not Smarties but pencils. The participant is then asked what a third person (to whom the contents have not been revealed) might think the Smarties tube contained. This requires the participant to reason out the beliefs of another person, and in this case the false belief of another. Some theorists suggest that thoughts such as these have to be encoded in language because of the embedded and serial nature of the reasoning – corresponding to (X thinks [Smarties in container]). Other modes of representation such as visual imagery do not seem to have the capacity to handle the embedded nature of such reasoning.

Theorists who advocate a propositional account of such reasoning differ in their views on the nature of the propositional code that is evoked. Carruthers (1998) and Siegal (1998) suggest that the code is that of natural language ('natural' here means languages such as English, French or Cantonese), and that natural language can be used both publicly for interpersonal communication, and intrapersonally through inner speech to mediate thinking. Pinker (1994) suggests that the medium of propositional thought is not natural language, but an abstract 'language of thought', or 'Mentalese'. Mentalese would be the operating language within the highest level of three-tier lexical processing models (e.g. Butterworth, 1989), with concepts being the lexicon of the language. The nature of grammar of Mentalese is far from certain and it is not clear how the characteristics of such a system can be determined by empirical investigations. The issue of redundancy in mental processes is again pertinent, as advocacy of Mentalese means that the human mind would operate with at least two internal propositional systems (natural language and Mentalese).

While it is not at all clear how an abstract language such as Mentalese might be scientifically investigated, it is possible to test the claim that certain types of thinking involve natural language propositions. The performance on theory of mind tasks of individuals who experience severe agrammatic aphasia might provide some insight into the role of grammar in some forms of thinking. It is critical in any test that the severity of the grammatical disorder is such as to impair both the understanding and production of propositional language (i.e. sentence constructions involving arguments linked by a predicate). Many individuals with agrammatic aphasia are able both to understand and construct simple propositions and thus, just as simple or 'proto-language' propositions may support public language, they may also support intrapersonal use of language in cognition.

The case of SA, a fifty-year old retired police sergeant with severe agrammatic aphasia, was reported in Varley (1998). Four years prior to the study he developed a subdural empyema in the left sylvian fissure. This resulted in severe agrammatic aphasia, and also a severe apraxia of speech. SA had relatively intact lexical processing, particularly in comprehension. A test of written lexical retrieval produced a score of 24/60 (PALPA 54 picture-naming test: Kay, Lesser and Coltheart, 1992). Speech output consisted of single element utterances, which were usually nouns. Evaluation of grammatical processing indicated a severe impairment of performance across all processing modalities. Scores on spoken and written sentence–picture matching tests (PALPA 55 and 56) were at chance (auditory 23/60, written 13/30). Impaired comprehension of verbs was indicated by chance performance on a verb semantics test (PALPA 57). Writing typically consisted of single element output – usually nouns and adjectives. When pressed to construct sentences, SA either produced strings of nouns and adjectives (e.g. 'woman red egg sekonda marriage'), or pseudo-grammatical constructions where content words were linked by grammatical words (e.g. 'woman a white as glass the red').

Despite these severe aphasic impairments, particularly in the area of grammar, SA appeared as one who had a disorder specific to language. In terms of activities of daily living, he was able to drive and he took responsibility for certain household chores. He was extremely resourceful in communication. He had communicative intentions which he sought to convey through flexible use of writing, drawing and gesture. In addition, he spent much of his time playing chess and other games with both human and computer opponents. Such games appear to require mentalistic understanding (of the opponent's plans and intentions) and strategic thinking in terms of one's own moves. In functional activities, SA appeared clearly capable of theory of mind-type reasoning despite a severe impairment of natural language grammar.

SA's ability to perform theory of mind reasoning was tested in an experimental setting using first-order false belief tasks. In a series of experiments, SA was presented with a familiar container (e.g. a pill bottle) which contained an unexpected content (e.g. buttons). The contents were revealed to SA, but not to a third person seated in the room. SA was then asked two questions: a false belief question ('What does X think is in the bottle?') and a reality question ('What is really in the bottle?'). Twenty theory of mind trials were completed following training on the linguistic content of the test questions, and SA scored significantly above chance at

18/20 (for a trial to be scored as correct, both the reality and false belief questions had to be answered correctly).

In a further series of tasks assessing other forms of reasoning, SA again showed intact performances. A test of causal reasoning was developed where SA was presented with an 'event' picture (e.g. a car crashed into a tree) and then asked to select from a choice of three pictures the likely cause of the event (e.g. 'alcoholic drink', 'axe' and 'helicopter'). At least one of the foils had a strong non-causal associative link to the event picture (tree–axe, car–helicopter). On this test, SA achieved a perfect score (15/15). The final task was selected from the Wechsler Adult Intelligence Scale (Wechsler, 1981). The Story Arrangement test requires a participant to arrange a series of line drawings into a sequence that tells a sensible story. Responses are both timed and scored for accuracy. SA achieved a score of 16/20 on this test, which places him on the 91st percentile of a normal age-matched population. The Story Arrangement test requires novel reasoning involving sequencing and cause and effect. SA's performance on this task was impressive.

What are the implications of these results for hypotheses regarding the role of grammar and propositional forms in human thought? The evidence provided by SA suggests that explicit language propositions are not involved in the types of reasoning demanded by the experimental tasks. The implicit-explicit knowledge distinction may be an issue here. The measures of grammatical ability that have been completed by SA are explicit measures, in that they tap conscious offline performance. In contrast to explicit measures, implicit tasks evaluate behaviour in unconscious or online tasks. An example of an implicit grammatical processing task is given by Tyler (1992). In a word-shadowing task, the participant is asked to listen for a particular word and to press a button as soon as they hear it. The implicit and unconscious element of the task is to vary the context leading up to the target word. If this context is grammatically well-structured and the participant is able to process grammatical structure, there should be a facilitation of the speed of the word identification judgement. If the preceding context is not grammatically well-structured, then there will be no such facilitation of the recognition judgement. The performance of SA on such tasks would be useful in order to clarify the issue of whether he has grammatical knowledge available to him at some level. If he has limited grammatical knowledge at an implicit level, it would be reflected in a lack of difference in response times to word targets in grammatically well structured or grammatically unstructured environments. In the absence of such evidence, we have to restrict our conclusion to proposing that explicit use of grammar is not a necessary component in the reasoning tasks. The results suggest that a natural language propositional code is not necessary for thought, although advocates of other propositional codes such as Mentalese might claim that the evidence from SA supports their position. They might ascribe his intact reasoning to retained Mentalese, despite disruption of natural language. There is nothing in the data that can disprove such an argument, but the Mentalese hypothesis might be discarded for other reasons, such as a reduplication of propositional codes and the difficulty in empirically testing the hypothesis.

What can be said, in summary, of our knowledge of the relationship between language and thought? The evidence from aphasic disorders is relatively sparse, and only a very small sub-group of aphasic people can provide data to contribute to the debate. These are individuals with profound impairments of lexical-semantic knowledge, or severe agrammatic disorders, or both. If an aphasic individual retains sufficient language ability to support some language function, this residual ability will be available for both interpersonal and intrapersonal use. The small amount of evidence that is available indicates that explicit use of grammar is not necessary to formulate even those thoughts that have an embedded nature. This evidence rests on a single case (SA) and needs to be replicated. With regard to the role of the lexicon, the notion of modality-specific semantic stores and distributed semantic representation would permit the aphasic person with disruption of lexical-semantic knowledge, assuming that damage was relatively specific to this store, still to be able to represent information mentally for purposes of intrapersonal cognition. If, however, damage extended across semantic stores, there would be more serious cognitive consequences.

We are now in a position to return to the view of the role of language in cognition outlined at the beginning of the chapter. The cognitive view, which suggests that language is central to human thought, is not supported by the evidence from aphasia. Does this then suggest that we should accept a communicative view of language – i.e. the view that language is used only for the purposes of interpersonal communication – or does the compromise supra-communicative view that language scaffolds human cognition appear viable. The communicative conception seems to deny the introspective evidence that there are times when we think things through in inner speech. These are often times of high cognitive load, for example when we are planning an essay or trying to resolve conflicting ideas. It is as though inner speech acts as a inner workspace, just as paper and pen can be co-opted as additional external workspace when the elements of the problem become too difficult to hold in memory. Adding phonological, orthographic or diagrammatic form to ideas makes them more memorable, and once in that form, they can be modified, combined or transformed. Language-mediated problem-solving is not restricted to verbal problems. Visual-spatial problems can also be assisted by inner speech support, as the intermediate steps towards the solution can be encoded and stored in language form. This supra-communicative view of language is well established in developmental psychology, where language is seen as scaffolding the acquisition of new skills (e.g. Vygotsky, 1934). Berk (1994) reported that children who talked themselves through novel tasks were the ones who were quickest to solve the problem. Dennett (1991) and Clark (1998) suggest that the possession of language has augmented the capacity of the human mind in ways that allow it to solve new classes of problems. Both Dennett and Clark suggest that the brain has a massive parallel processing architecture, which enables fast and simultaneous processing of different signals. Language has enabled an additional serial or sequential processing capacity within the human mind. A supra-communicative view of the relation between language and cognition, while not proposing that inner speech sentences constitute thoughts, would suggest that a language impairment, of whatever severity, robs the problem-solver of an important cognitive tool. Some of the evidence of impaired performance of aphasic individuals on apparently non-linguistic problems may potentially be accounted for in this way (e.g. Whitehouse, Caramazza and Zurif, 1978; Cohen, Kelter and Woll, 1979; Semenza, Denes, Lucchese et al., 1980; Caramazza, Berndt and Brownell, 1982; Wayland and Taplin, 1982).

The issues of language and its interrelationships with thought at times appear theoretical and abstract. But there are practical implications for such issues. A fundamental justification for providing rehabilitative services to people with aphasia is that these individuals still have communicative intentions and are able to formulate messages or coherent thoughts that they wish to convey to others. Other issues, such as the right of the aphasic person to make a will, to provide testimony to a court of law, and to make decisions regarding his or her future, are based on the assumption that rational thinking and reasoning abilities are in place.

Knowledge and executive functions

In the previous sections we have examined the role of lexical-semantic knowledge in overall conceptual knowledge. We have also addressed the question of the form of the reasoning that is involved in apparently sequential and embedded theory of mind tasks. We have suggested, on the basis of data from study of a single case, that explicit natural language grammar does not appear necessary for even this class of thoughts. We have also claimed that the distributed nature of total conceptual knowledge (e.g. across different sensory-perceptual systems) allows, in the case of focal damage, for the possibility of residual knowledge sustaining conceptual activities. There is also recognition, from a supra-communicative stance, that a language impairment may rob an individual of an important crutch to cognition. In this final section, the question to be addressed is whether it is possible to have a largely intact conceptual knowledge base, but to be unable to use it in strategic ways, for example, in a piece of novel reasoning.

There are two patient groups that we shall discuss in this section: those with 'dysexecutive syndrome' following lesions of the prefrontal cortex, and patients with vascular lesions of the non-language dominant hemisphere (usually the right). Both groups of patients are generally described as having intact language ability, particularly at the levels of grammar and lexicon, although abnormal discourse and conversational structure is commonly reported in this patient group (e.g. Perkins, Body and Parker, 1995). The abnormalities in communication can be seen as a result of disruption of cognitive processes that are interlinked with language, rather than a result of a primary language deficit (e.g. Hagen, 1981), although some investigators into right-hemisphere communicative disorders in particular, maintain that the linguistic disruptions are a result of primary and specific language impairments (e.g. Myers, 1999). Damage to the prefrontal cortex may result from a variety of conditions, but one of the most common causes is closed head injury (CHI) that results from road traffic accidents, falls and blows. The right-hemisphere damaged (RHD) group are usually seen as a distinct clinical population from CHI, but McDonald (1993) points to similarities in the cognitive and communicative profiles of the two groups. McDonald goes on to suggest the similarity of features may stem from a common pathology: CHI patients often have bilateral prefrontal cortex lesions; while the RHD group may have more focal damage to the right prefrontal cortex.

Patients with prefrontal cortex damage often perform well on tasks which tap well-learned knowledge and skills. On a picture-naming task, for example, a patient's performance may not be significantly different from normal. However, when the same individual is given a lexical task that requires a strategic search of lexical-semantic memory – e.g. a verbal fluency task such as 'Recall the names of as many animals as you can in 90 seconds' – performance is often surprisingly discrepant to that of control subjects and to expectations based on picture-naming performance. Although both picture-naming and verbal fluency tasks tap lexical-semantic processing, the strategic element of the verbal fluency task becomes necessary once the first group of highly frequent and highly prototypical category members have been recalled. Subsequent retrieval is best organized by sub-categories, such as farm animals, domestic pets, and types of ape. The yield of a strategy has to be monitored and when it is about exhausted a switch to a new strategy is required. There are also memory components within the task – remembering which items have been retrieved already so that there is not perseveration of responses. Patients with lesions to the prefrontal cortex may produce a small number of set members, often with perseverations of previous items, and an absence of clustering of responses into groups such as 'monkey, gorilla, chimpanzee, baboon', indicating that search strategies are not being utilized. Behavioural difficulties are not restricted to lexical-semantic tasks. Many abilities, including activities of daily living (e.g. Shallice and Burgess, 1991), are impaired as a result of the difficulty with planning, and strategy implementation.

The development of models of the cognitive functions involved in novel and strategic tasks is difficult, simply because of the complexity of the behaviours that such models attempt to explain. These behaviours are often grouped together under the label of 'executive functions' (and hence the disorder 'dysexecutive' syndrome). An 'executive' is something that has oversight and governs a range of units or departments. In cognitive terms, the executive is something that monitors and regulates other processing modules, such as language, or visual perception. This notion fits well with the observation that patients with prefrontal cortex lesions do well on tasks in which the individual modules can complete using their well learned routines (such as picture naming), but begin to show impaired performance on tasks that impose additional or novel demands. A widely used model of executive function is that of Norman and Shallice (1980). This model is not uncontroversial – for example, Dennett doubts whether such a mechanism is psychologically plausible (1991, 1998) – but it has proved productive as a descriptive model in guiding both research into and the management of dysexecutive disorders. Norman and Shallice suggest that much of ongoing behaviour is controlled by schemata, learned patterns of behaviour that have been built up through previous experiences. Incoming sensory information triggers a particular schema, which in turn generates an appropriate behavioural response. The disturbing experience of driving along a well-known route and suddenly realizing that you have no recollection of the last ten miles is an illustration of how appropriate behaviour patterns are triggered automatically in response to environmental stimuli (presumably you successfully navigated your way around all the obstacles in your path). Schemata are not, however, available for all situations. In some instances we might be faced with a novel task for which no schema is available. Alternatively, the usual 'auto-pilot' ways of responding to inputs might be resulting in failure. One such example is performance on stroop tests (Stroop, 1935). In the classic stroop test a subject is presented with a colour word (e.g. *blue, red*) printed in a colour of ink which is incongruent with the word (*blue* printed in green ink, for example). The usual way to respond to words is by their verbal content. If you are asked to read a word list, you call out the words and not a perceptual characteristic such as the type of font or the colour of the ink the word is printed in. In a stroop task, subjects respond to a word list by the perceptual features, thus the word list is reported by colour while verbal content has to be ignored. This requires the inhibition of the automatic behavioural schema. Norman and Shallice suggest that in such situations behaviour is controlled by an executive component – the 'supervisory attentional system' (or SAS). To this point, the model of cognition outlined by Norman and Shallice is not overly controversial, but the difficulties really begin when one attempts to specify how the SAS might work. (How does it monitor the performance of other systems? How does it take a controlling role in behaviour? How does it generate a novel plan?)

Despite the difficulties, an important element of the SAS model is the distinction between ongoing behaviour triggered by external stimuli and a form of behavioural control that is less tied to the environment. Baddeley (1992) elaborates a model of working memory within which the model of the SAS can be accommodated. Working memory involves the capacity to sustain mental representations. The model developed by Baddeley focuses on phonological representations (sustained in the phonological loop of the working memory model) and visuo-spatial representations (maintained in the visuo-spatial sketchpad). Phonological working memory allows inner speech representations to be maintained (rather as one silently repeats a telephone number over and over in your head while you search for a pencil with which to write it down). But phonological working memory does not just represent a passive store of information. These internal speech forms can be manipulated and operated upon in order to transform information. For example, a task such as alternately retrieving alphabet letters and numbers (1-A-2-B-3-C- . . .) represents this type of transform function. There is a clear link here to the supra-commu-nicative view of language with which we began this chapter. Working memory represents a processing system which can operate with a number of codes, one of which is inner speech. It can operate as an internal workspace to support cognitive activities such as problem-solving and behavioural planning. Instead of solving problems by trial and error, we can run virtual simulations of solutions in our minds, without running the risk of embarking on action which may lead to a costly failure. Investigations of the brain localization of working memory function suggest that both the left and right prefrontal cortices play a significant role. This evidence comes from neuropsychological studies of the effects of lesions of the prefrontal cortex and from measures of brain activation during working memory tasks (Smith and Jonides, 1994; McCarthy, Blamire, Puce et al., 1994). An individual with a prefrontal lesion may as a consequence have a deficit in the operating system of working memory, despite an intact inner speech code. In contrast, a patient with a profound language disorder resulting from lesion of the peri-sylvian cortex in the language-dominant hemisphere may lose one of the codes with which working memory operates. Other codes, for example, visuo-spatial representations, may be spared, together with much of the operating system of working memory. This differential impairment of functions may account for how an individual with profound aphasia may still be capable of sustaining complex strategic thinking (such as defeating an opponent at chess), while an individual with seemingly intact language can fail on tasks that involve even small degrees of strategic thought, such as word fluency.

Conclusion

In this chapter, we have addressed issues that concern how language operates intrapersonally, rather than the more usual and obvious public and interpersonal use of language. A supra-communicative view of language suggests that it can support other cognitive operations and a speech-based code, operating within phonological working memory, may be important in scaffolding performance on a range of both language and non-language tasks. In addition, certain ideas might be very difficult to entertain without language mediation, particularly ideas about abstract entities that may lack representation outside of the language system. I have, however, also argued for a distributed knowledge base, with our integrated sense of a concept being in fact the consequence of fluid coalitions of distributed knowledge. In this way, destroying an entire concept, particularly of a highly imageable object, may not occur in instances of focal brain damage. This results in the possibility of the individual with brain damage still retaining a rich mental life following injury, even in the face of profound public disabilities.

References

Baddeley AD (1992) Is working memory working? The Fifteenth Bartlett Lecture. Quarterly Journal of Experimental Psychology 44A(1): 1–31.

Beauvois MF (1982) Optic aphasia: a process of interaction between vision and language. Philosophical Transactions of the Royal Society of London B298: 35–47.

Berk L (1994) Why children talk to themselves. Scientific American, November: 78–83.

Bub DN, Black S, Hampson E, Kertesz A (1988) Semantic encoding of pictures and words: some neuropsychological observations. Cognitive Neuropsychology 5: 27–66.

Butterworth B (1989) Lexical access in speech production. In W Marslen-Wilson, (Ed) Lexical Representation and Process. Cambridge, MA: MIT Press.

Caramazza A, Berndt R, Brownell H (1982) The semantic deficit hypothesis: perceptual parsing and object classification by aphasic patients. Brain and Language 15: 161–89.

Carruthers P (1996) Language, Thought and Consciousness: An Essay in Philosophical Psychology. Cambridge: Cambridge University Press.

Clark A (1998) Magic words: how language augments human computation. In Carruthers P, Boucher J, (Eds) Language and Thought: Interdisciplinary Themes. Cambridge: Cambridge University Press.

Cohen R, Kelter S, Woll G (1979) Conceptual impairment in aphasia. In Bauerle R, Egli U, von Stechow A, (Eds) Semantics from Different Points of View. Berlin: Springer Verlag.

Dennett DC (1991) Consciousness Explained. New York: Little Brown Co.

Dennett DC (1998) Reflections on language and mind. In Carruthers P, Boucher J, (Eds) Language and Thought: Interdisciplinary Themes. Cambridge: Cambridge University Press.

Garrett M (1982) Production of speech: observations from normal and pathological language use. In Ellis A (Ed) Normality and Pathology in Cognitive Functions. London: Academic Press.

Hagen C (1981) Language disorder secondary to closed head injury: diagnosis and treatment. Topics in Language Disorders 1: 73–87.

Howard D, Orchard-Lisle VM (1984) On the origin of semantic errors in naming: evidence from the case of a global aphasic. Cognitive Neuropsychology 1: 163–90.

Howard D, Patterson KE (1992) The Pyramids and Palm Trees Test. Bury St Edmunds: Thames Valley Test Co.

Kay J, Lesser R, Coltheart M (1992) Psycholinguistic Assessment of Language Processing in Aphasia. Hove: Lawrence Erlbaum.

Kertesz A (1988) Cognitive function in severe aphasia. In Weiskrantz L, (Ed) Thought without Language. Oxford: Oxford University Press.

Kertesz A, Lesk D, McCabe P (1977) Isotope localisation of infarcts in aphasia. Archives of Neurology 34: 540–601.

Levelt WJM (1989) Speaking: From Intention to Articulation. Cambridge, MA: MIT Press.

McCarthy G, Blamire AM, Puce A, Nobe AC, Bloch G, Hyder F, Goldman-Rakic P, Shulman RG (1994) Functional magnetic resonance imaging of human prefrontal cortex activation during a spatial working memory task. Proceedings National Academy of Sciences USA 91: 1233–40.

McCarthy RA, Warrington EK (1988) Evidence for modality-specific naming systems in the brain. Nature 334: 428–30.

McDonald S (1993) Viewing the brain sideways? Frontal versus right hemisphere explanations of non-aphasic language disorders. Aphasiology 7: 535–49.

Myers PS (1999) Right Hemisphere Damage Disorders of Communication and Cognition. London: Singular.

Norman D, Shallice T (1980) Attention to action: willed and automatic control of behaviour. In Davidson R, Schwartz G, Shapiro D (Eds) Consciousness and Self-Regulation: Advances in Research and Theory. New York: Plenum.

Paivio A, Yuille JC, Madigan SA (1968) Concreteness imagery and meaningfulness values for 925 nouns. Journal of Experimental Psychology Monograph Supplement 76(2): 1–25.

Perkins M, Body R, Parker M (1995) Closed head injury: assessment and remediation of topic bias and repetitiveness. In Perkins M, Howard S, (Eds) Case Studies in Clinical Linguistics. London: Whurr.

Pinker S (1994) The Language Instinct. London: Penguin Books.

Saffran E (1982) Neuropsychological approaches to the study of language. British Journal of Psychology 73: 317–38.

Semenza C, Denes G, Lucchese D, Bisiacchi P (1980) Selective deficit of conceptual structures in aphasia: class versus thematic relations. Brain and Language 10: 243–48.

Shallice T, Burgess PW (1991) Deficits in strategy application following frontal lobe damage in man. Brain 114: 727–41.

Siegal G (1998) Representing representations. In Carruthers P, Boucher J, (Eds) Language and Thought: Interdisciplinary Themes. Cambridge: Cambridge University Press.

Smith EE, Jonides J (1994) Working memory in humans: neuropsychological evidence. In Gazzaniga MS (Ed) The Cognitive Neurosciences. Cambridge, MA: MIT Press.

Stroop J (1935) Studies in interference in serial verbal reactions. Journal of Experimental Psychology 18: 643–62.

Tyler LK (1992) Spoken Language Comprehension. Cambridge, MA: MIT Press.

van Mourik M, Verschaeve M, Boon P, Paquier P, van Harskamp F (1992) Cognition in global aphasia: indicators for therapy. Aphasiology 6: 491–99.

Varley R (1998) Aphasic language, aphasic thought: an investigation of propositional thinking in an a-propositional aphasic. In Carruthers P, Boucher J, (Eds) Language and Thought: Interdisciplinary Themes. Cambridge: Cambridge University Press.

Vygotsky L (1934)) Thought and Language. Translated by Kozulin, 1962: reprinted 1986. Cambridge, MA: MIT Press.

Warrington EK (1975) The selective impairment of semantic memory. Quarterly Journal of Experimental Psychology 27: 635–57.

Warrington EK, Shallice T (1984) Category specific semantic impairments. Brain 107: 829–53.

Wayland S, Taplin J (1982) Nonverbal categorization in fluent and nonfluent anomic aphasics. Brain and Language 16: 87–108.

Wechsler D (1981) Wechsler Adult Intelligence Scale – revised. San Antonio: The Psychological Corporation.

Whitehouse P, Caramazza A, Zurif E (1978) Naming in aphasia: interacting effects of form and function. Brain and Language 6: 63–74.

CHAPTER 10

Two subsystems for semantic memory

WENDY BEST

This book began with an overview of models of semantic memory. These models have been re-visited throughout the book. This chapter proposes a model of semantic memory with two separate but inter-connected meaning systems. It will become clear that the ideas presented here have their foundations firmly in previous models of semantic memory and owe much to the consideration of neuropsycho-logical data. The aim is to propose a model that is clinically as well as theoretically motivated and which can inform thinking about break-down and rehabilitation.

To introduce the chapter we shall consider three phenomena that can arise following brain damage, which need explanation in relation to disruption to a normal system of semantic memory. Firstly, there are the category-specific semantic deficits reviewed in detail in Chapter 4: in these cases people will perform better with particular semantic categories – e.g. non-living things – than with others – e.g. living things. Models must be able to account for both this and the reverse dissociation (superior perform-ance on non-living things) together with the patterns of performance on related tasks. Secondly, there is the contrast between damage to verbal meanings found in aphasia, and the wider damage to meanings found in dementia (see Chapters 7 and 8). Finally, within aphasia, there is the general tendency for greater impairment on abstract/low imageability items found across a variety of tasks (e.g. Coltheart, Inglis, Cupples et al., 1998; Franklin, Howard and Patterson, 1994, 1995; Nickels and Howard, 1995). Again, however, models need to be able to be damaged to show the reverse, more unusual, pattern of superior performance with abstract words (Breedin, Saffran and Coslett, 1994; Marshall, Pring, Chiat et al., 1996; Warrington, 1975). We shall return to each of these issues later in this chapter.

Distributed object concepts

We begin by considering an influential model proposed by Allport (1985; see Chapter 1, this book, Figure 4). In this model, meanings are represented by auto-associated patterns which are distributed across different attribute domains. For example, the representations for 'necklace' will be distributed over visual, kinaesthetic, tactile and action orientated elements. Key to the model is the claim that the elements that are involved in coding the sensory attributes of an object also form part of the patterns of activity which represent object-concepts in semantic memory.

Allport's model has a number of characteristics that make it appealing when attempting to account for patterns of breakdown following brain damage. In particular, concepts are held to be distributed over several domains and may therefore be less susceptible to brain injury than representations defined over single or fewer domains (such as word forms). So, for example, if there is damage to the visual elements, a partial representation for 'necklace' would still be sustainable as the auto-associated elements across intact domains, such as tactile and action orientated elements, will combine with the impaired information from the visual domain. This fits with the 'graceful degradation' of performance whereby knowledge does not appear to be lost entirely but where performance is partially impaired relative to normal functioning (for further data in support for this model, see Howard, Best, Bruce et al., 1995; Marshall et al., 1996).

This model makes the claim that multi-sensory/functional aspects of a concrete item can be co-activated to form a representation for that item. Although not explicitly discussed by Allport (1985), the model also entails overlapping patterns for items with similar meanings; thus the representation for 'kettle' would share action, tactile and visual elements with 'teapot'. If such a system were damaged, items that overlap those to which it is exposed would be likely to result in strongly related responses (e.g. naming a picture of a kettle as a teapot). These 'co-ordinate errors' occur, for example, in picture naming in both aphasia (see Chapter 5) and semantic dementia (Hodges, Graham and Patterson, 1995).

Beyond distributed object concepts.

While Allport's model is extremely useful in thinking about the meanings of single concrete objects, there are a number of aspects of knowledge that are difficult to incorporate within its framework.

Firstly, it is not clear how the many and varied associations between concrete concepts arise. For example, we know that oranges grow in hot countries, that babies sleep in cots, and that ginger can settle the stomach. Even these few examples of links between concrete concepts differ widely in the type and degree of association. One can speculate that some aspects of association may be available on the basis of visual meaning, so that we may visually link babies and cots (in the same way as other things that co-occur in the visual environment). There may also be some perceptual link between oranges and things associated with warmer climes – for example, we should be surprised to see oranges growing in British woodland. However the knowledge that oranges grow in hot countries seems likely to be held mainly within a verbal domain, along with much other encyclopaedic knowledge. Other associations between concrete objects are likely not to be visually coded but to rely entirely on learned links (ginger and stomach settling) which may well be learned verbally and perhaps coded also via links with Allport's kinaesthetic elements.

Secondly, it is difficult to envisage how the model represents abstract concepts that form a huge part of our meaning system and which themselves rest on a wide range of further meanings – such as 'life', 'freedom', 'time', 'family' – given that these concepts have few sensory or functional properties.

Finally, there is a big difference between people with aphasia and people with semantic dementia which is not captured by attributing both deficits to damage to a distributed sensory/functional meaning system. To return to the example of 'kettle', a person with aphasia, with an acquired language problem, would not, *unless they had accompanying deficits*, mistakenly put a teabag in a kettle – even though they might mistakenly call a kettle a teapot. In contrast, in later stages of semantic dementia object concepts are impaired (see Chapter 8 for further discussion). The extent to which visual and verbal knowledge are disrupted in semantic dementia varies from person to person (Hodges et al., 1995; see also Lauro-Grotto, Piccini and Shallice, 1997, footnote 2). The picture is not entirely clear because some people with semantic dementia have much worse comprehension with verbal than non-verbal materials (e.g. IW: Lambon Ralph and Howard, 2000) and some people with aphasia demonstrate poor performance on tasks with picture input (Chertkow, Bub, Deaudon et al, 1997). However, the aim here is to see the wood and not the trees: many people with aphasia appear not to have impaired non-verbal semantic knowledge, and people with semantic dementia may demonstrate impaired knowledge even when presented with real objects in situations where no language is required.

Two subsystems for semantic memory

In response to these limitations an alternative model is being proposed which encompasses verbal and non-verbal semantic subsystems. These subsystems together form a whole semantic system. They differ from one another, however, in terms of processing and the nature of the representations. Both abstract concepts and the abstract associations between concepts are represented in a verbal semantic subsystem. This is linked with the distributed sensory/functional representations for object concepts. The model is illustrated in Figure 1. While associations between items in this model are coded in the verbal semantic subsystem, this does not preclude the existence of some types of association within the sensory/functional system. For example, the representations for items that are commonly seen or used together may co-activate one another to an extent.

The system of 'object concept semantics' here is the sensory functional distributed model of Allport (1985). This system is organized by category to the extent that semantic co-ordinates will have overlapping auto-associated meaning patterns.

The connected subsystem labelled 'verbal semantics' codes linguistic meaning for both concrete and abstract concepts. This will result in dual coding (Paivio, 1986) for some aspects of the meaning of concrete objects. The strengths of Paivio's dual coding hypothesis and problems with the original model are discussed in Chapter 1. While there is duplication, the aspects of meaning representations that occur in both the object concept

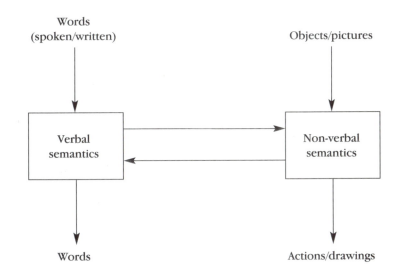

Figure 1. Two intercommunicating semantic subsystems: the verbal subsystem is accessed from words and mediates spoken and written language production. The non-verbal subsystem is accessed from non-verbal modalities of input (vision, touch, etc.) and is used to mediate action. Accessing the full meaning representation for a concrete concept necessitates activation across both semantic subsystems.

and verbal semantic subsystems will differ and the extent to which dual representation occurs is open to further investigation. An example may help illustrate this point; while I 'know' that a wombat has legs (perhaps by inductive reasoning: Howard, 1985), I do not have a (readily available) visual form for these.

In contrast, abstract concepts are more likely to be represented verbally – though we are able sometimes to create visual images for specific abstract concepts these are likely to be fairly individual and will not generally be present for most items. The verbal system is organized according to semantic category but this organization is abstracted away from the sensory patterns on which the conceptual representations were based in development.

Both the occurrence of category co-ordinate semantic errors (see Chapter 5) and the very existence of category-specific deficits (see Chapter 4) point to categorical organization of verbal semantics. Consideration of the development of meaning systems is beyond the scope of this chapter. However, recent research points strongly to the importance of object shape in driving object naming in young children, and to the increasing influence of object function in attributing object names with age (Landau, Smith and Jones, 1998).

Related models of semantic memory

The suggestion that there are two (or more) semantic subsystems, and that some aspects of meaning are coded in different ways, is far from new, and it might be noted that the figure above bears a strong resemblance to Figure 5 in Chapter 1, and to Figure 12.5 in Shallice, 1988. However, this model differs from that proposed by Shallice in that his model does not rely on the distributed form/function representations proposed by Allport (1985) for object concept knowledge.

In the model proposed here, functional and sensory aspects of meaning are both part of one auto-associated pattern. In early versions of the model, Warrington and Shallice (1984) make a distinction between these sensory and functional aspects of meaning in order to account for semantic category-specific disorders (see also Chapter 4, this book; Farah and McClelland, 1991 – described in detail in Chapter 2 of this book; Saffran and Schwartz, 1994). In practice, however, the distinction may be blurred between those models with separate sensory and functional subsystems and Allport's distributed model, which spans these domains. Further understanding relies on implementation of different models and our ability to make sensible links between the results of such modelling and normal and neuropsychological data.

There is considerable debate about the nature of visual and verbal semantic systems, in particular focusing on whether the systems have different modalities of input or representation (Caramazza et al., 1990; Coltheart et al., 1998; Shallice, 1987, 1988; Warrington and Shallice, 1984). This debate is fuelled by case studies of people with striking modality-specific effects. For example, Kartsounis and Shallice (1996) describe a person with a 'modality-specific memory loss' where performance was impaired only from visual input (with good performance from verbal input). In this case the 'modality' referred to is 'modality of input'. There are echoes of earlier papers, and Shallice's conception of visual and verbal semantic subsystems appears to entail duplication of information within these semantic subsystems, each accessed by a different modality.

The model presented in this chapter does not entail complete duplication of semantic information: verbal and non-verbal object representations differ. In the model proposed here the *same* information can be accessed from words and from objects although each will have more direct links with the system of meanings that matches the modality of presentation. For example, on *hearing* the spoken word *ball* both verbal and sensory/functional information can be activated. However, the route to sensory/functional aspects of meaning is via linguistic meaning. On *seeing* (an object which is recognized as) a ball, both sensory/functional and verbal information can be activated. However, in this case, the route to verbal meanings is via the distributed non-verbal meaning system. Damage may disrupt either the meaning subsystems or the links between these systems. Clear and testable predictions arise from these claims. Also, such a model can account for the classic pattern in dysphasia of impaired understanding/expression of verbal meanings (particularly for abstract items) while sensory/functional meanings can remain intact; there is damage to the verbal semantic subsystem but no damage to object concept semantics.

One piece of evidence commonly used to support models with a unitary amodal semantic system (see Chapter 1) is item consistency across tasks tapping semantic knowledge from different modalities of input (over and above the consistency predicted on the basis of other underlying variables: Lambon Ralph, Howard, Nightingale et al., 1998; Lambon Ralph and Howard, 2000). While such consistency can be parsimoniously explained with respect to a single system, it is also compatible with a system with verbal and non-verbal subsystems. If, for example, there is damage to non-verbal object concept representations, this will impair performance regardless of the modality of input used to tap the impaired knowledge. Likewise, an impaired verbal subsystem will disrupt performance on any task requiring this knowledge. In summary, damage to either subsystem will result in item consistency across modality of input and the pattern of performance will depend on the exact demands of the task and the extent of damage to representations.

The two subsystems proposed in this chapter are *not* the sensory and functional subsystems proposed in other models (e.g. Farah and McClelland, 1991). Also, the model does *not* entail separate storage of semantic knowledge for words and pictures. This is a common interpretation of the meaning of the term 'modality-specific semantic system'. (See Chapter 1 for discussion, and Lambon Ralph and Howard (2000) as an example of authors who interpret the term in this way.) In the model proposed here, both words and pictures access the same meaning subsystems, albeit in different ways.

Finally, in relating this model to other conceptualizations of semantics we turn to Bierwisch and Schreuder (1992) who argue for a distinction between linguistic and extra-linguistic determinants of meaning. For example, in contrasting 'He left the institute an hour ago' with 'He left the institute a year ago', *institute* and *leave* have different meanings – i.e. 'a building' and 'a change of location', as opposed to 'an organization' and 'a change of affiliation'.

A further relevant point clearly made by these authors is that, out of context, many utterances are ambiguous, emphasizing the fact that our meaning representations for a message are richer than the linguistic expression we either hear or produce. The simple model proposed here to deal with the meaning of individual items may be extended to allow for wider representations of meaning. At this level also, there appears to be evidence for both verbal and non-verbal meaning subsystems.

In summary, the model put forward in this chapter incorporates two linked subsystems. The non-verbal subsystem represents meanings in the way proposed by Allport (1985). The meaning of an item *is* the auto-associated pattern distributed across sensory and action orientated domains. This non-verbal system is linked to a verbal subsystem that codes aspects of meaning which may not be captured by the non-verbal sensory/functional patterns such as associations between items. In particular, the meaning of abstract concepts will be coded in this subsystem. The *complete* meaning for a concrete concept is fully achieved only when representations in *both* subsystems are active. Thus, part of our semantic memories are closely tied to the mechanisms of perception and motor output, as suggested by Allport (1985) and part of our semantic memories, probably in different areas of the brain, are abstracted away from these domains. These subsystems *together* provide a full representation of meaning.

Relating category-specific semantic deficits to the model

Studies of people with category-specific deficits have been influential in driving the specification of models of semantic memory (e.g. Coltheart et al, 1998; Caramazza and Shelton, 1998). In Chapter 4 of this book such studies were reviewed and, from studies investigating attribute knowledge, two particular patterns of deficit emerged. In the first, there are people with a category-specific deficit for living things who demonstrate impaired knowledge of sensory and functional attributes for living things, without impairment on attribute judgements for non-living things (EW: Caramazza and Shelton, 1998; DB: Lambon Ralph et al., 1998; Laiacona, Barbarotto and Capitani, 1993; Laiacona, Capitani and Barbarotto, 1997). A tentative suggestion, in relation to the model presented here, is that there is a deficit focused in the 'living things' area of the categorically organized verbal semantic subsystem. This hypothesized impairment suggests two further lines of investigation. Firstly, testing with non-verbal materials should reveal *relatively* unimpaired sensory functional knowledge on tasks where no *verbal* input/output/associative knowledge is required. Secondly, testing of verbal associations/encyclopaedic knowledge (e.g. country of origin, life-span, habitat, etc.) would be predicted to be relatively impaired in relation to living things.

A finding which does not fit in a straightforward way with this account is the impairment in drawing which can co-occur with this deficit (e.g. for DB: Lambon Ralph et al., 1998). However, it was DB's drawing to dictation that was impaired, i.e. a task mediated by input from (impaired) verbal semantics. Straight copying remained intact. In contrast, delayed copying, which may with known objects rely to some extent on holding the visual form and word meaning, was impaired and tended to show 'regression to the mean' for animals or semantic errors for both living and non-living things (e.g. bat → bird, sword → pin, helicopter → plane. Also of relevance here is the fact that DB suffered from Alzheimer's type dementia, suggesting damage distributed throughout meaning and other cognitive systems (see Chapter 7). While most of the damage may fall within the verbal semantic system, other areas are unlikely to be wholly intact.

The second pattern that has been found is damage to knowledge of sensory attributes across semantic categories, i.e. regardless of whether items are living or non-living (AC: Coltheart et al., 1998; IW: Lambon Ralph et al., 1998). IW, who suffered from semantic dementia, also demonstrated a small category-specific deficit for non-living things once stimuli were well controlled. How might this pattern of performance relate to the model presented here? The most obvious claim would be that the focus of the damage is the visual elements of the distributed object concept semantic subsystem. This would tailor well with IW's impaired drawings, which tend to have missing features but retain elements of associative knowledge. For example, her 'bat' is drawn upside down, her sword has a sharp point, her duck (possibly) has feathers. In a more recent paper about work with IW, Lambon-Ralph and Howard (2000) emphasize the contrast between her comprehension of words (which is severely impaired) and of pictures (which is superior). An account of this, in relation to the present model, would have to postulate damage to lexical representations (input or output or lexical semantic), in addition to the impairment within the non-verbal subsystem already proposed to explain her poor recall of sensory attributes. The suggestion of multiple deficits is compatible with the progressive nature of her problem. The claim is also supported by AC's improved performance on answering visual attribute questions with pictures present. (See Chapter 4 for detailed discussion of AC's performance.)

Finally, how might the model be damaged to account for the performance of SE (Moss, Tyler and Jennings, 1997; however, see Laws, Evans, Hodges et al., 1995), who appeared to have a semantic deficit restricted to the visual properties of living things? As semantic co-ordinates have overlapping auto-associated meaning patterns in the model, this deficit might be the result of damage to a restricted part of the visual elements in the object concepts subsystem, that which contains the patterns for living things. SE showed particularly poor performance for the distinctive visual properties, which might be especially vulnerable to damage as they do not share auto-associated elements with other aspects of meaning. An alternative hypothesis is that SE has damage to pre-semantic structural descriptions and that the category-specific effect is not real but 'falls out' of this level of impairment. (See the section on pre-semantic representations below.)

Specifications to be made

A key aspect of the model here is the distinction between verbal and non-verbal knowledge. Several aspects of the model remain underspecified. However, it is common to envisage models as able to be specified in more detail in a number of different ways (Shallice, 1993) and this should not stop us from evaluating the broad framework of a model.

Verbal semantics

The nature of the verbal semantic system is open to debate. Within the field of psychology, models tend to involve a list of propositions or 'meaning postulates' (Howard, 1985). Similarly, the OUCH model outlined in Chapter 1 is held to incorporate perceptual and action knowledge within an amodal system (Caramazza, Hillis, Rapp et al., 1990). The fact that we can provide a list of attributes when asked about meaning may make this an appealing account but does not necessarily reflect the way linguistic meanings are organized.

One important consideration concerns the lexical specificity of representations within the verbal semantic system. The tentative claim made here is that verbal concepts can map directly in a 1:1 relation to lexical items used in language in comprehension and production. It should be clear, however, that the major claim of this chapter, that there are semantic subsystems for sensory/functional and for verbal knowledge, does not rest upon the nature of the representations in the verbal system.

Within the verbal system it is likely that concrete concepts will generally entail more semantic features (however these are represented) than abstract concepts (Plaut and Shallice, 1993). Thus, when the system is damaged abstract concepts are likely to be relatively more impaired. Furthermore, the representations for concrete items will receive support from intact sensory/functional representations. Such support will not be available for more abstract items. Effects of imageability in the predicted direction have been found across a variety of tasks including reading (in deep dyslexia, Coltheart et al., 1980), comprehension (Franklin et al., 1994) and picture naming (Franklin et al., 1995; Nickels and Howard, 1995).

However, there are exceptions to this general pattern. For example, CAV (Warrington, 1975) was able to read abstract items better than concrete items. In a more recent study, Marshall et al. (1996) worked with RG, who had semantic jargon aphasia. RG had a tendency to use abstract rather than concrete words and this was reflected in his performance on comprehension tasks which tended to be better with abstract items (see also Breedin et al., 1994). In addition, RG was better at naming from abstract definitions – e.g. a fortified historic building – than concrete definitions – e.g. a building with turrets and a drawbridge. The authors relate their findings to Allport's (1985) model and claim that RG has a deficit in the visual domain of the semantic system. How can RG's deficit be interpreted with respect to the model presented here, where there is held to be dual coding of some information in the verbal and sensory/functional semantic subsystems? One possibility is that RG has damage both to the visual elements within the object semantic subsystem and to concrete items within the verbal semantic subsystem. The fact that his pattern of performance is relatively unusual might fit with this interpretation. An alternative is that, as the authors claim, the deficit is in the visual elements

of object concepts, and that the verbal representations alone are not sufficient to support naming.

It should be noted that RG's performance on naming to abstract definitions was not at ceiling (56% correct, compared with 32% correct in
response to concrete definitions for the same items). This is in line with
either of the above possibilities. RG may have an impairment in both
semantic subsystems, but the extent of the damage is asymmetrical.
Alternatively, the pattern of performance could suggest damage to only
one system but that information from *both* subsystems is necessary to
support naming.

Thus, in modelling semantic memory, it is important to demonstrate
how a system might be damaged to result in both 'normal' and reverse
concreteness effects. (See Plaut and Shallice's 1993 model of oral reading,
and Chapter 9 of this book.)

The nature of the link between subsystems

Central to all processing that involves words and objects concepts is the
link between verbal and non-verbal meaning. The nature of this link is not
specified here. One possibility, discussed in relation to RG (Marshall et al.,
1996) is that, in many tasks, the meaning of a concept that spans both
semantic subsystems is activated in its entirety. Thus the 'auto-associa-
tions' that occur in the distributed sensory/functional domain also 'auto-
associate' with verbal knowledge. In this case the verbal semantic
subsystem would form another part of an entire meaning system.

There is a fine line between the notion of a single semantic system
distributed over different domains and the two subsystems proposed in
this chapter. In particular, an amodal system with 'privileged access'
according to modality of input (e.g. OUCH, outlined in Chapter 1) may be
difficult to distinguish from a model with closely linked subsystems. Both
models require further specification. However, the evidence for unidirec-
tional disruption between different subsystems (as found in optic aphasia
and discussed below) is hard to reconcile with a single amodal system.
Additionally, within a unitary system one presumes that all the knowledge
that we have about an item is activated each time the concept is active,
whereas this may not necessarily be the case in the model presented here.
Our understanding of such issues will be furthered by increasing the specification of models (e.g. by implementing them) and by better controlled
investigation of normal and disrupted semantic processing (see Chapter 4).

Actions and verbs

The focus of this chapter is the nature of semantic representations for
objects. Here we shall consider briefly the possible nature of the represen-

tations for actions within the different subsystems with the aim of clarifying some of the claims that are being made. (For further discussion of this and related issues readers are referred to Chapter 3.) Taking the concrete action of pouring as an example, consider first the non-verbal representation. This might encompass a range of concepts of pouring actions with different visual exemplars, different hand grasps, etc. The auto-associated pattern of activity for this action would link directly to the representation in the verbal subsystem, which is abstracted away from the specific sensory/functional forms of the action to an idealized more abstract cluster of pouring events with a particular focus. The properties represented here will include the semantics of the verb such as the number and nature of the thematic roles. Finally, there are direct links from this level to the individual lexical item *pour* and to its syntactic properties held at the level of the lemma. (See the section below on the relationship between this model and models of speech production.)

The representations in conceptual and verbal semantics may have different boundaries with the verbal representations relating in a much more straightforward way to individual lexical items.

Relationship with other models of object/word processing

It is beyond the scope of this chapter to discuss the wide range of possible ways in which the model proposed might relate to other aspects of processing (such as episodic memory or syntactic knowledge). However, we shall consider its relation to two areas relevant to other parts of this book.

Pre-semantic representations

Firstly, we shall consider evidence for the existence of separable pre-semantic stores in which modality-specific forms are represented, which can be used for recognition. An example of such a store is the structural descriptions system proposed by Humphreys and Riddoch (1987). The existence of such a store does not sit easily with Allport's (1985) idea that the very patterns of activation that occur with a particular input *are* the concept representations. However, the existence of cases with intact performance on tests of object decision combined with poor performance on tests of object knowledge (e.g. IW: Lambon Ralph et al., 1998) suggests the functional separation of the representations used to perform the two types of task.

This issue remains to be clarified by studies with tighter methodology. In particular, it was argued in Chapter 4 that damage to a structural descriptions system will result in *apparent* category-specific deficits on visually presented tasks, due to the nature of visual representation across semantic categories – i.e. the greater perceptual overlap between exemplars from categories of living things (Humphreys, Riddoch and Quinlan, 1998). This argument may account for what is occurring in the case of AC (Coltheart et al., 1998), and is termed the 'visual explanation' of category-specific deficits.

Models of speech production

Recent models of speech production argue for a level of representation, referred to as the 'lemma'. (The meaning of this term is not entirely clear and has changed with time: contrast Levelt, 1989, with Levelt, Roelofs and Meyer, 1999. See also Chapter 9 of this book.) The important point here is that it is a level of representation between semantic memory and phonological representations (Levelt et al., 1999). Indeed, in the model proposed by Levelt et al., the semantic features comprising an item are stored in memory which is used to access a 'lexical concept representation' which maps directly to the 'lemma'. The 'non-decomposed' lexical concept representation contrasts with decomposed semantic representations proposed by other theorists (e.g. Bierwisch and Schreuder, 1992).

In contrast, in another influential and implemented model of speech production (Dell, 1986, 1989; Dell, Schwartz, Martin et al., 1997) word nodes are linked directly with semantic feature nodes. These models differ in a number of other important ways. For example, in the model of Levelt et al. the activation feeds forward through the system; in contrast, the model of Dell et al. involves interactive activation between levels.

How might the model proposed in this chapter relate to these models of speech production? Restricting the discussion to levels of representation, the semantic features of Dell's model might form part of the verbal semantic subsystem proposed here. Thus there could be a fairly straightforward mapping between the two proposals in terms of levels of representation.

In contrast, the model proposed here would entail one fewer level of representation than that proposed by Levelt et al. (1999). In their model, the task of naming a picture would involve processing involving at least the following representations: visual semantic; verbal semantic (decomposed); lexical concept (non-decomposed lexically-specific semantic representations); lemma; phonological form. Whether there is evidence for such a range of representations is open to further debate. (For evidence from different types of anomia, see Nickels, in press.)

The verbal semantic subsystem proposed here would link directly to a lexical level of representation (such as the lemma level proposed by Levelt et al., 1999). It would therefore reduce by one the number of levels of representation required in picture/object naming; there is no requirement for the additional 'lexical-concept' level between semantics and lemma.

Evidence in line with two subsystems

We shall end this chapter with a brief overview of the evidence, detailed elsewhere, in favour of separate verbal and non-verbal (sensory/functional) semantic subsystems.

a) The existence of modality-specific aphasia, in which objects can be named to definition but not from visual presentation (e.g. optic aphasia: Campbell and Manning, 1996; Lhermitte and Beauvois, 1973). A recent example is provided by Druks and Shallice (1996). The person they worked with could name items from definition but not from vision or touch. They found access to semantic representations from visual and verbal stimuli was equally good and suggest, therefore, that the deficit was in the links between visual and verbal semantic subsystems. Such cases are particularly striking as there are good reasons to expect superior performance with visual over verbal input on many tasks (Lambon Ralph et al., 1997).

b) The contrast between aphasia and semantic dementia. In some people with aphasia there may be damage solely to relatively peripheral language systems such as those used for repetition. However, in most people with aphasia there is damage to lexical and meaning systems. For example, the same pattern of breakdown can occur with spoken and written words, suggesting there are problems central to meaning rather than with access to meaning (e.g. CJ: Franklin, 1989). In general, however, people with aphasia – in the absence of other deficits – appear to demonstrate good knowledge of object meaning and function where words are not involved (Chertkow et al., 1997). This contrasts with the pattern of performance shown in late-stage semantic dementia, in which people become unsure what items are and what they are used for (Funnell, 1995). This broad contrast between the two types of disorder reflects the distinction between verbal and sensory/functional semantic subsystems, although in the latter case both systems may be damaged.

c) Within the context of a single categorically organized semantic system, it is difficult to explain the existence of deficits where there is damage to knowledge of sensory attributes across semantic categories (e.g. AC: Coltheart et al., 1998; IW: Lambon Ralph et al., 1998).

d) The fact that different languages parcel up world meanings differently may also be used to support the claim that there are separate non-verbal and verbal semantic subsystems. (See Chapter 3 for related discussion.) The assumption here is that speakers of different languages (at least from similar cultures) will have similar non-verbal subsystems that are generated from experiences with the real world. Speakers of different languages will share boundaries in the sensory/functional system while having different boundaries between items in the verbal system. This argument is not straightforward, however, as it taps into basic questions of whether language can influence our perceptions and representations of the world, questions that have themselves generated huge amounts of research.

e) The repeated finding of better performance on concrete than abstract items may stem from the fact that concrete items may have more 'features'. However, in this model it may also arise from the dual coding (verbal and non-verbal) of some aspects of the meaning of concrete items.

While clinicians with experience of working with people with different types of breakdown might think that the distinction between conceptual and linguistic semantic systems is patently obvious, in many recent models this distinction is not made (e.g. Caramazza et al., 1990; Farah and McClelland, 1991; Riddoch et al., 1988 – outlined in Chapters 1 and 2 of this book). In order to make progress in understanding how meaning is structured, how this can break down, and ways in which damage may be remediated, we need a broad framework. The fundamental distinction between verbal and non-verbal conceptual knowledge should not be ignored.

Outstanding questions

1. Can implemented models of semantic memory be lesioned so as to result in patterns of performance commonly and uncommonly shown in people with brain damage?
2. As investigations of semantic memory impairments are refined to look further at knowledge of features, will additional patterns emerge that will help specify this or other models of semantic memory?
3. How are associations between concepts coded in semantic memory, and how is this knowledge best tested? For example, many items in the Pyramids and Palm Trees Test (Howard and Patterson, 1992) may be completed correctly on the basis of straightforward visual co-occurrence (e.g. associating 'baby' with 'cot' and 'curtain' with 'window'). Other items, however, require different types of associative knowledge to be available (e.g. associating 'stethoscope' with 'heart', 'caterpillar' with 'butterfly'). In particular, the relationship between performance on this frequently employed task and the nature of semantic impairment needs further refinement. Many people with aphasia perform

within normal limits on the 'three picture' version of this test, showing impairment only when written words are used (e.g. TC: Nickels, 1992). This might suggest a problem restricted to verbal semantic and/or to lexical processing. However, other people with aphasia are impaired even on the 'three picture' version, suggesting wider semantic involvement.

4. How does the nature of the deficit interact with the information required in a task and the nature of information made available in the task. For example, a problem with activating full auto-associated patterns for object concepts might be alleviated in tasks using visual input. The missing information may be partly reinstated by provision of the visual form. Similarly in using attribute questions one may actually be priming knowledge that has been partially impaired.

5. Can rehabilitation studies further inform our understanding? For example, will treatment focusing on a particular attribute type generalize across semantic categories? This outcome might be predicted by a model of the type proposed in this chapter but not by a model with a single amodal semantic system. Of course, such studies will be constrained by the appropriateness of treatment and the nature of a person's semantic deficit. However there is clearly scope for therapy to inform theory, and vice versa.

Conclusion

This chapter has proposed the existence of two linked semantic subsystems: verbal and non-verbal (sensory/functional). The latter is held to be distributed over several sensory domains in the manner proposed by Allport (1985). The former entails verbal meaning representations for concrete and abstract items and the associations between items. While the model remains considerably underspecified, the basic framework can accommodate the main patterns of performance found in category-specific semantic disorders and superior performance on concrete over abstract items often found in aphasia. The fact that some people with aphasia have difficulties with word meanings while maintaining intact non-verbal concepts provides further support for the model's structure. Future models of semantic memory would benefit from taking account of the evidence for two subsystems of meaning.

References

Allport DA (1985) Distributed memory modular subsystems and dysphasia. In Newman SK, Epstein R, (Eds) Current Perspectives in Dysphasia. Edinburgh: Churchill Livingstone. pp 32–60.

Bierwisch M, Schreuder R (1992) From lexical concepts to lexical items. Cognition 42: 23–60.

Breedin SD, Saffran EM, Coslett HB (1994) Reversal of the concreteness effect in a patient with semantic dementia. Cognitive Neuropsychology 11: 617–60.

Campbell R, Manning L (1996) Optic aphasia: a case with spared action naming and associated disorders. Brain and Language 53: 183–221.

Caramazza A, Hillis AE, Rapp BC, Romani C (1990) The multiple semantics hypothesis: multiple confusions? Cognitive Neuropsychology 7: 161–89.

Caramazza A, Shelton J (1998) Domain-specific knowledge systems in the brain: the animate-inanimate distinction. Journal of Cognitive Neuroscience 10: 1–34.

Chertkow H, Bub D, Deaudon C, Whitehead V (1997) On the status of object concepts in aphasia. Brain and Language 59(2): 203–32.

Coltheart M, Inglis L, Cupples L, Michie P, Bates A, Budd B (1998) A semantic subsystem of visual attributes. Neurocase 4: 353–70.

Coltheart M (1980) The semantic error: types and theories. In Coltheart M, Patterson K, Marshall J, (Eds) Deep Dyslexia. London: Routledge and Kegan Paul.

Dell GS (1986) A spreading activation theory of retrieval in sentence production. Psychological Review 93: 283–321.

Dell GS (1989) The retrieval of phonological forms in production: tests of predictions from a connectionist model. In Marslen-Wilson W (Ed) Lexical Representation and Process. Cambridge, MA: MIT.

Dell GS, Schwartz MF, Martin N, Saffran WM, Gagnon DA (1997) Lexical access in aphasic and non-aphasic speech. Psychological Review 104: 801–38.

Druks J, Shallice T (1996) CHECKA modality linked naming impairment and multiple-semantics. Brain Cognition 32(2): 273–76.

Farah MJ, McClelland JL (1991) A computational model of semantic memory impairment; modality specificity and emergent category specificity. Journal of Experimental Psychology: General 120: 339–57.

Franklin S (1989) Dissociations in auditory word comprehension: evidence from nine 'fluent' aphasic patients. Aphasiology 3: 189–207.

Franklin S, Howard D, Patterson K (1994) Abstract word meaning deafness. Cognitive Neuropsychology 11: 1–34.

Franklin S, Howard D Patterson K (1995) Abstract word anomia. Cognitive Neuropsychology 12: 549–66.

Funnell E (1995) Objects and properties – a study of the breakdown of semantic memory. Memory 3(3–4): 497–518.

Hodges JR, Graham N, Patterson K (1995) Charting the progression in semantic dementia – implications for the organisation of semantic memory. Memory 3(3–4): 463–95.

Howard D (1985) The semantic organisation of the lexicon: evidence from aphasia. Unpublished PhD thesis. University of London.

Howard D, Best W, Bruce C, Gatehouse C (1995) Operativity and animacy effects in aphasic naming. Special issue in honour of Ruth Lesser. European Journal of Disorders of Communication 30: 286–302.

Howard D, Patterson K (1992) Pyramids and Palm Trees. Thames Valley Test Company. Bury St Edmunds: UK.

Humphreys GW, Riddoch MJ (1987) On telling your fruits from your vegetables – a consideration of category specific deficits after brain damage. Trends in Neurosciences 10(4): 145–48.

Humphreys GW, Riddoch MJ, Quinlan P (1988) Cascade processes in picture identification. Cognitive Neuropsychology 5: 67–103.

Kartsounis LD, Shallice T (1996) Modality specific semantic knowledge loss for unique items. Cortex 32: 109–19.

Laiacona M, Barbarotto R, Capitani E (1993) Perceptual and associative knowledge in category specific impairment of semantic memory: a study of two cases. Cortex 29: 727–40.

Laiacona M, Capitani E, Barbarotto R (1997) Semantic category dissociations: a longitudinal study of two cases. Cortex 33: 441–61.

Lambon Ralph MA, Howard D (2000) Gogi aphasia or semantic dementia? Simulating and assessing poor verbal comprehension in a case of progressive fluent aphasia. Cognitive Neuropsychology.

Lambon Ralph MA, Howard D, Nightingale G, Ellis AW (1998) Are living and non-living category specific deficits causally linked to impaired perceptual or associative knowledge? Evidence from a category specific double dissociation. Neurocase 4: 311–38.

Lambon Ralph MA, Graham KS, Patterson K, Hodges JR (1997) Is a picture worth a thousand words? Evidence from concept definitions by patients with semantic dementia. Brain and Language.

Landau B, Smith L, Jones S (1998) Object perception and object naming in early development. Trends in Cognitive Sciences 2: 19–24.

Lauro-Grotto R, Piccini C, Shallice T (1997) Modality-specific operations in semantic dementia. Cortex 33: 593-622.

Laws KR, Evans JJ, Hodges JR, McCarthy RA (1995) Naming without knowing and appearance without associations: evidence for constructive processes in semantic memory? Memory 3: 409–33.

Levelt WJM (1989) Speaking: from Intention to Articulation. Cambridge, MA: MIT Press.

Levelt WJM, Roelofs A, Meyer AS (1999) A theory of lexical access in speech production. Behavioural Brain Sciences 22: 1–38.

Lhermitte F, Beauvois MF (1973) A visual-speech disconnection syndrome: report of a case with optic-aphasia, agnosic alexia and colour agnosia. Brain 96: 695–714.

Marshall J, Pring T, Chiat S, Robson J (1996) Calling a salad a federation: an investigation of semantic jargon, Part 1 – Nouns. Journal of Neurolinguistics 9: 237–50.

Moss HE, Tyler LK, Jennings F (1997) When leopards lose their spots: knowledge of visual properties in category specific deficits for living things. Cognitive Neuropsychology 14: 901–50.

Nickels LA (1992) The autocue? Self-generated phonemic cues in the treatment of a disorder of reading and naming. Cognitive Neuropsychology 9: 155–182.

Nickels LA, Howard D (1995) Aphasic naming: What matters? Neuropsychologia 33: 1281–1303.

Nickels LA (in press) Words fail me: symptoms and causes of naming breakdown in aphasia. In Rapp B (Ed). Handbook of Cognitive Neuropsychology.

Paivio A (1986) Mental Representations: A Dual Coding Approach. Oxford: Oxford University Press.

Plaut D, Shallice T (1993) Deep dyslexia: A case study of connectionist neuropsychology. Cognitive Neuropsychology 10(5): 377–500.

Riddoch MJ, Humphreys GW, Coltheart M, Funnell E (1988) Semantic systems or system? Neuropsychological evidence re-examined. Cognitive Neuropsychology 5: 3–25.

Saffran EM, Schwartz MF (1994) Of cabbages and things; semantic memory from a neu-
    ropsychological perspective – a tutorial review. In Umilta C, Moscovitch M, (Eds)
    Attention and Performance 15: Conscious and Nonconscious Information
    Processing. Cambridge, MA: MIT Press. pp 507–36

Shallice T (1987) Impairments of semantic processing: multiple dissociations. In
    Coltheart M, Sartori G, Job R, (Eds) The Cognitive Neuropsychology of Language.
    London: Lawrence Erlbaum Associates.

Shallice T (1988) From Neuropsychology to Mental Structure. Cambridge: Cambridge
    University Press.

Shallice T (1993) Multiple semantics: whose confusions? Cognitive Neuropsychology
    10(3): 251–61.

Warrington EK (1975) The selective impairment of semantic memory. Quarterly
    Journal of Experimental Psychology 27: 635–57.

Warrington EK, Shallice T (1984) Category specific semantic impairment. Brain 107:
    829–54.

CHAPTER 11

Understanding Meanings

KAREN BRYAN, JANE MAXIM AND ALISON CONSTABLE

We have carefully used the term 'semantic processing' in the title of this book, but the study of semantic processing is dogged by the use of terms that refer to aspects of this processing. 'Semantic memory' can be precisely described (as in Chapter 1) but can also be used to refer to the semantic system, which is less defined. Similarly, a term such as 'semantic representation' can have different meanings in different research papers. There is a need to be precise at the same time as attempting to try to reconcile aspects of semantic processing into a coherent whole, which would allow us to understand how semantic processing occurs in normal individuals.

Semantic processing in the human brain is undoubtedly vastly more complex than our understanding of it and our ability to describe it. Semantic processing is complex, variable, adaptable and even compensatory in certain individuals, in certain circumstances. It may be unreasonable to expect to find one model which is compatible with a wide variety of findings to explain all this – yet it is this that we need in order to progress to greater understanding of the semantic system and its architecture.

In models of semantic processing, we must be able to incorporate aspects of normal variation such as, for example, the effects of gender – is female semantic processing the same as male? Are there contextual effects on semantic processing – for example, do we alter our processing of meaning depending on who we are talking to? There is ample evidence to show that people use a different range of grammatical structures, intonation patterns and non-verbal information in different linguistic contexts and with different conversational partners (see Couper-Kuhlen and Selting, 1996; Coupland and Jaworski, 1997, for discussion) and there is some evidence that the linguistic expression of meaning is also subject to this variation (Cheshire, 1982; Gardner-Chloros, 1997). Semantic

241

processing is influenced by such features but current psychological models do not generally reflect these influences. Fodor (1998), for example, argues that current ways of thinking about concepts need a radical overhaul.

Other influences such as concreteness, abstractness, frequency, familiarity and many others have been more systematically investigated (see previous chapters). A definitive model would have to be able to deal with each of these factors and combinations of them. The idea of factors carrying different 'weights' is attractive and somewhat concrete and pictorial, but simple addition or subtraction of weights begins to look too simplistic. What determines the weights to be added and under what criteria?

Funnell (in Chapter 1) has outlined the different approaches to modelling semantic memory, but we do not yet have what could be described as a definitive model. The models vary in their ability to explain different types of pathological data, which is not surprising when one takes into account the fact that different models have been developed to explain different types of normal and pathological data. Even when a model is able to account for all the available data, it is sometimes difficult to see how the validity of the model can be established. Models should be able to predict outcomes as well as explaining data from experimental and clinical studies if we are to move forward in understanding the dynamics of the semantic system. In addition, models need to address how such a system actually operates in different people under different circumstances. For example, factors such as idiosyncratic differences, choice of certain strategies in certain circumstances and preferred modes of operation may be very salient when people use semantic information in everyday tasks. We know that such factors are worthy of consideration as other areas of research indicate that there may be very significant differences between 'laboratory' findings and findings from studies of more functional and contextual tasks. For example, there are many reports of older people having problems with verbal memory, but longitudinal studies show that normal older people do not have problems remembering salient information in their daily life (Cavanaugh, 1983).

The model needed, therefore, may depend upon a series of interconnected issues and questions, of which the following are typical.

- What question is being asked?
- What data will be applied?
- What theoretical hypothesis is being tested?
- What individual and contextual factors will influence semantic processing?

A particular model may be appropriate to answer the above questions in terms of research methodology, but the assumptions underlying the questions may have influenced the resulting model. For example, the OUCH model of semantic memory outlined in Chapter 1 (Caramazza, Hillis, Rapp et al., 1990) has been used to explain a range of deficits in participants with Alzheimer's disease, but it is not so easy, however, to use the theory to explain the preservation of personally salient information in semantic dementia. OUCH suggests that there is one semantic system which is accessed via different input and output processes. What specific processes would have to be damaged to selectively spare personally salient information? One answer might lie in the input and output processes themselves which, hypothetically, could work better for information in constant use over time.

There are also areas of semantic memory that are not addressed by models which are primarily designed to explain pathological processing arising from damage to the brain. For example, how do children acquire semantic memory in the first place? An increasing body of conceptual knowledge is acquired by children as their experience of the world increases. The lexical labels that represent this knowledge are acquired gradually, along with other lexical information about how words sound and the functions they fulfil in connected speech. As new items are added and concepts refined, the lexicon expands and becomes increasingly intricate, and children's abilities to both understand and convey meaning grow.

Of course, semantics is much more than the meanings of single words. We also have to consider meaning relations within multi-word utterances (as discussed in Chapter 4), along with the complexities of constructing and decoding meaning within discourse. Here semantic development becomes intricately entwined with that of syntax and pragmatics.

Models of speech and language processing that can account for the complexities of language development are relatively few. Those that do exist may include 'semantics' or 'semantic representations' (e.g. Stackhouse and Wells, 1997).

There might be justification for leaving aside learning as part of development when it comes to a semantic processing model, but learning does not stop at a particular point in the lifespan. There is no evidence for a decline in vocabulary size as people get older and very elderly people are able to acquire new vocabulary and to use words to express new shades of meaning (Salthouse 1988), for example, in the current use of 'cool' to denote a positive quality rather than a substance which is no longer warm. Thus learning and adaptation of knowledge need to be incorporated into the model of semantic processing.

What we need next is to reconcile the necessary features from each type of model to form a coherent model that can illustrate all aspects of semantic processing and explain different types of data. This might be an unrealistic idea but there are developments which may indicate that such a model might be forthcoming before too long:

- Work on network models of semantic memory (see Chapter 1) which allow different aspects of the processes involved to be utilized to accomplish a range of tasks.
- Connectionist models (described in Chapter 5) allow complex networks to be operated under 'different' conditions and to be 'lesioned' in different ways. Such models may allow modelling to become more efficient and less fractionated. Alternatively, this may be an unrealistic expectation of technology.
- Models which have separate conceptual and verbal semantic systems (such as that proposed in Chapter 10) appear to go further towards accounting for the wide variety of patterns of semantic breakdown.

Although we don't yet have a definitive model of semantic processing, the principle of referring to a model to guide assessment and understanding of deficits has influenced clinical practice. The application of cognitive neuropsychological modelling to the assessment of aphasia has radically altered assessment and has allowed therapeutic intervention to be targeted, hypothesis-driven and monitored (Byng and Black, 1996). Such approaches have influenced research-driven practice for some time and are becoming more widespread among practitioners in relation to aphasia although not so routinely used in relation to other disorders such as language difficulties associated with dementia.

Application of what might be termed 'pathological' data to models of semantic processing is important as error data must be explained by the model (as discussed by Levy in Chapter 5). Similarly models should not give rise to types of errors that do not occur in certain naturally occurring conditions. Plaut and Shallice (1993), for example, explore whether computation modelling can account for language deficits and the process of remediation, concluding that their model learned in a way that suggested a different approach to remediation from that in the research literature.

However, there is a danger that semantically based therapy may be used without convincing evidence for a theoretical basis to the deficit. For example, children with specific language impairment who have lexical difficulties (difficulties in learning and in using lexical items) often present with word-finding problems. Traditionally, therapy for word-finding difficulties has involved semantic elaboration work without the necessary evidence that semantic problems are the cause of the individual child's difficulties. Bishop (1997) reviews all the possible causes of word learning difficulties in children, and suggests that problems with conceptual development and phonological processing may be involved. What may be suggested by therapy studies in these children (Constable, Stackhouse and Wells, 1997; McGregor, 1994) is that semantic knowledge, its organization, and its usage can be compromised by difficulties in other aspects of speech and language processing. A similar situation is found in adults with acquired semantic problems, for example, those associated with aphasia. In Chapter 2, Nickels discusses the fact that in some cases what is termed 'semantic therapy' is not actually aimed at remediating semantic processing itself, but may have, for example, the aim of improving word-finding skills.

Work on semantic theory has influenced semantic therapy, and vice versa. Chapter 2 describes work on semantic category deficits, which have received much attention in the research literature. The difficulties and ambiguities in interpreting data from such studies illustrate a number of areas where aspects of semantic processing interrelate. For example, visual effects need to be distinguished from other semantic effects – but meaningfully related objects often share visual similarities, e.g. tyre and wheel. Familiarity is an important variable but is difficult to dissociate from other semantic factors in order to produce carefully controlled material for research studies. Work on dissociations in clinical cases between living and non-living items is a case in point: such items will vary on other parameters such as familiarity, so that alternative interpretations of data may be possible.

Another factor which must be considered in relation to studies of semantic processing is the use of normative data. Normative data need to be representative, with age and level of education being important factors. However other issues may be relevant: for example, Holland (1990) asks what norms are appropriate for judging language disordered patients in long-term residential units. Here, factors such as opportunity, context and staff expectations would be relevant, and would cast doubt on the use of data from age-matched but community-living older people.

Studies also need to resolve possible tension between the need to develop tests that all (or at least a wide range of normal people) can reliably perform and the need for norms that are not restricted to a ceiling effect which makes comparison to normal performance statistically problematic. Clinicians may opt for tests where normal performance is at ceiling, in order to show reliably that even a small number of errors indicates a deficit, or at least a performance level requiring further investigation, whereas researchers may seek norms that are not at ceiling (see Chapter 2).

Hence, there is a call for well-controlled studies where parameters are tightly defined and semantic information is controlled. These studies are exactly what theoretical research needs, but when applied to patients with brain damage, such material can be criticized as too remote from the complexity of what occurs in normal processing. However, the semantic therapy studies described by Nickels in Chapter 6 show that carefully targeting therapy to the exact process that is damaged is essential in achieving measurable therapy effects. Studies such as Nickels and Best (1996a, 1996b) illustrate carefully targeted therapy that does address specific aspects of semantic processing. However, this in itself is not enough, and the authors describe the need to control factors such as exactly how the task is presented, and how feedback is included and/or presented in order to achieve success both within tasks and extending to generalization.

As Best outlines in more detail, we need to specify the semantic processing breakdown, detail the therapy, and control all of the compounding variables. Possibly this may be in order to exclude other factors interfering with the therapy effect, but it also creates the opportunity to allow deliberate manipulation of these factors to achieve success, for example by adding in feedback on performance if completing a task does not have a desired effect on outcome measures.

As more therapy studies emerge, it is possible to chart a number of well replicated semantic 'therapies' that can be manipulated to take into account the patient's exact deficits and preserved abilities. This has led to a repertoire of therapies to which Nickels refers in Chapter 5. A number of semantic therapies are also described in Byng, Swinburn and Pound (1999). But we need many more of these studies and we need to compare participants who have been tested and treated on the same materials so that cases can be compared. Comparison of cases would assist us in predicting who will benefit from which therapy, with specified control of confounding factors in order to achieve a positive outcome. It may be important to note here that studies replicating therapies are important, but perhaps less often published. Similarly, well-controlled theoretically-driven therapy studies which do *not* produce the 'desired results' also need to be published.

Work on the encoding of meaning in verbs as children learn language illustrates further complexities in semantic processing. With verbs there is not necessarily a one-to-one correspondence between a word and an event. Similarly, comparisons between languages show that events – for example, putting a cup down on a table – are not in a one-to-one relationship with linguistic forms. So, as language is learned, meaning is shaped by the forms and structures of the language (see Chapter 3).

Work on verb semantics in the acquired field is beginning to confirm that the structure of the language used by therapists and researchers in tests and therapy procedures may exert an influence on comprehension and use of verbs in therapy. Language structure may then be a compounding variable that requires control in any study of semantic processing. In relation to therapy, the possibility of deliberately manipulating language structure to influence or facilitate semantic processing arises and can begin to be investigated in a systematic fashion.

There may be parallels between how verb processing develops and how it breaks down, but there are inevitably other issues to consider. Contrasts between concrete, perceptually-based properties and more abstract, language-dependent properties may be important in distinguishing why some people with aphasia find verbs harder to process than nouns. The directness of mapping from meaning to (verb) forms and other semantic properties or features – for example, actions, states, and relationships between actors and instruments – may all influence whether a person with language impairment associated with aphasia can use and/or comprehend verbs.

Difficulties with verb processing do not equate with particular types or categorizations of aphasia, and the reverse patterns (greater difficulty with nouns than verbs) that have been described indicate that 'verb' problems cannot be explained as part of a syntactic deficit – we have to take account of meaning and the relationship between form and meaning.

Just as we are thinking about the relationship between aspects of language – phonology and semantics, syntax and semantics – we need also to consider the relationship between semantic language functions and other cognitive functions. Should language be considered as just 'one' form of general cognitive functioning, or is there something qualitatively different about language? (Varley discusses this question in more detail in Chapter 9.)

Another factor that has to be considered in relation to language breakdown associated with pathology is normal ageing. Studies of lexical knowledge suggest that the structure of semantic information is well preserved or even intact, but that access declines proportionally with age (Laver and Burke, 1993). Therefore word-finding difficulties associated with tip-of-the-tongue state are commonly described and are outlined in detail with explanatory theories in Chapter 6. What is perhaps less commonly recognized is that other aspects of language change as people age and that this change is not always negative. Indeed, there is evidence that discourse skills may improve, with greater elaboration and use of hierarchically detailed episodes being rated by listeners as more preferable and more memorable than narratives of younger people (Kemper, Rash, Kynette et al., 1990). This provides a challenge to ageist attitudes to ageing, where ageing is automatically equated with quantitative and qualitative detriments in performance!

However, other aspects of discourse processing in older people do conform to prevalent stereotypes. Older people may have difficulties with referential communication tasks, although methodologies must be examined carefully. As Kemper and O'Hanlon (Chapter 6) point out, in a task such as formulating labels for abstract drawings, where a finding is that older people do not elaborate the previous label but formulate a new one, the influence of factors such as memory difficulties (or even subtle limitations) must be considered. Also, factors such as reported verbosity and increased subject matter related to painful disclosures about illness, bereavement, and so on may reflect changes in underlying semantic functioning such as reduced inhibition. However, the influence of other factors cannot be ignored. Many older people have a reduced communication network that may give rise to loneliness, and hence verbosity in company may therefore be partly reactive to the opportunity. Negative life events may also be reflected in more negative topics of conversation. In older people, researchers tend to look for organic causes to support or explain such findings – in other words, a pathological cause. Styles such as 'verbose' may be used by younger people in certain circumstances. But this approach is not so prevalent in relation to younger people. So we expect (and even think it is advisable) for younger people to talk about negative experiences, to join self-help groups of similarly afflicted people, and even to seek professional counselling to maximize the positive power of talking about experiences. Here, psychosocial explanations are preferred and pathology is not so actively sought out.

Similarly, it is reported that older people are slower in relation to discourse processing, they extract less, and they have difficulties in processing syntactically more complex sentences. But studies that examine more functional and everyday activities do not report deficits. It is possible that some of the 'research experimental' findings are in fact reflecting very positive adaptations. So, slowing down in text processing may assist processing. Parsing into chunks may decrease the load on working memory if the material is complex, but this may lead to errors of integration of information. So the 'problems' may reflect real-world behaviours that lead to positive adaptation for everyday living. There may be some tension between the recognized need for highly specific studies of semantic processing which analyse out confounding factors and pinpoint aspects of processing, and those that take a more global view of the way in which people 'normally' process semantic information.

Work on semantic processing in dementia has to face the same type of methodological issue. Here, psychosocial factors such as disuse and lack of opportunity need to be distinguished both from normal language change associated with ageing and from pathological changes in other areas of cognition which may impact on language such as memory and orientation.

Again, the value of detailed assessment and of consideration of preserved abilities as well as deficits has proved important. People with semantic dementia are frequently misdiagnosed: direct assessments of word comprehension and naming, and face and object recognition, are needed for diagnosis, along with careful case history taking to reveal the typical pattern of preserved abilities in relation to deficits (see Chapter 8). Correct diagnosis is important since the management of these patients differs from that of patients with Alzheimer's disease. Anticholinergic medication for AD is inappropriate in these people, and behavioural management can be tailored to their needs. Using a person's preferred routines and incorporating care provision within their existing routine will make such care more useful to a person with semantic dementia. There is evidence that new learning can take place if it is personalized and if it allows the person to utilize preserved autobiographical memory. Idiosyncratic strategies can also be understood and maximized – for example, the lady described in Chapter 8, who 'shops' by matching empty packets with new ones on the shop shelves, is compensating very well, and a system to routinely keep old packets and incorporate them into the shopping routine might be useful. Many of the so-called 'problem' behaviours can be understood if the disorder of semantic processing is understood.

Chapter 8 discusses the clinical potential that has emerged from the understanding of semantic dementia, and the routine testing of language processing and, more specifically, semantic processing is advocated. Here is an example of clinical practice lagging behind research findings. Unfortunately, people with dementia do not routinely have their dementia type diagnosed and therefore do not routinely have their semantic processing (or even possibly any other aspect of their language processing) assessed. They may present at a memory clinic or a specialist care of the elderly service that has a speech and language therapist or a clinical psychologist, where the primary focus is diagnosis and where the available professional expertise does not extend to advising on how to support a deteriorating semantic system.

Even in relation to Alzheimer's disease there is research to show that access to the semantic system can be increased (at least in the early- to mid-stage of the disease). The necessity for early assessment of language in people with dementia – using appropriate materials, procedures and an adequate timescale – is a particular need for clinicians. Tests should also minimize the processing load on other skills such as working memory and visual processing. Many research assessments, while suitable for research, are not suitable for people who are frail or have poor attentional resources, and are anyway too long for the constraints within which most health care providers work.

A group of clinicians who work with people with dementia are currently working on a minimum data set of tests, for clinical use to assess language in people with dementia, that has norms developed by the group (Bryan, Binder, Funnell et al., 1999). Initiatives such as this will hopefully enable more clinicians to assess people with dementia on a routine basis, and will allow both clinicians and researchers to identify people who present with unusual profiles which indicate a need for further assessment.

As dementia progresses, language may decrease, although communicative potential is always there. A very sensitive study by Hamilton (1994) showed that detailed analysis of conversations between the researcher and a woman with advanced dementia could still achieve meaning. Meaning might not always be fully established, and the researcher increasingly bore the responsibility for sustaining the conversation but information was exchanged and both participants gained satisfaction from this.

In other situations language may remain relatively intact, but communication is disrupted by severe difficulties in output. Here, the dissociations between performance in one area compared to another are found. Varley (in Chapter 9) describes a person with severe expressive aphasia who could drive, play chess and function on a daily basis, as well as being very resourceful with ways to convey information, such as drawing.

Dissociations of functions are important, since therapeutic possibilities may arise where one relatively well preserved function can be used to compensate for another, This may be highly specific – for example, using a picture to replace a written word to facilitate word retrieval – or more general – for example, in validation therapy, where the ability to produce language is used to support memory and orientation in people with dementia to enhance emotional well-being (Feil, 1992).

This raises the issue of how language is built into thought, and how the two develop and then retain and update a meaningful semantic system (as well as other facets of cognition) when access in or out is so severely restricted. Essentially this is a version of the 'language and thought' debate – how does one function when the other is impaired?

Varley (in Chapter 9) outlines three broad approaches to the role of language in other areas of communication. Language can be seen as entirely separate from thought and conceptual knowledge; language may be seen to have a central role in cognition; or a compromise, supra-communicative view is possible, where language is seen as separate from cognition, but capable of scaffolding or supporting certain internal cognitive functions such as planning (via inner speech). Varley makes a case for the latter, with the implication that a language impairment would rob an individual of a tool for operating certain other cognitive functions. There is also ample evidence from studies of people with Alzheimer's disease and semantic dementia that the semantic system can deteriorate in isolation from, or at different rates to, other cognitive functions and other levels of language processing.

The relationship between language and other cognitive skills is being explored in a number of fields where language difficulty may affect other cognitive processes (which are disordered), or it could be argued that language disorder may be a more direct causal factor in the cognitive difficulty (Tager-Flusberg, 1991). In other words difficulty in using language may underlie some other aspects of processing. The relationship between semantic processes per se, and pragmatic processes – in terms of usage of language in context for a communicative purpose – is another area of research where advances still need to be made.

In children with so-called semantic-pragmatic disorder (Bishop, 1997) the relationship between semantic difficulties and pragmatic difficulties is contentious. Is it possible that these children have difficulty with pragmatic aspects of interaction because their semantic understanding is not fully developed? It is debatable whether such children have specific language impairment or whether their difficulties relate to more fundamental underlying processing difficulties (Boucher, 1998). There are difficulties in investigating such questions because of a lack of relevant standardized measures for semantics and the need for a naturalistic context in assessment (Mogford-Bevan and Sadler, 1992).

Whatever the nature of the disorder might be in semantic-pragmatic disorder or in autism, what is increasingly recognized is the value of systematic and individualized psycholinguistic investigation of children presenting with speech and language difficulties (for example, Constable, Stackhouse and Wells, 1997).

In schizophrenia, Frith (1997) suggests that the problems lie in communication rather than language itself, and that the communication difficulties arise from an inability to mentalize so that the beliefs and intentions of others are not correctly recognized. Theory of mind tests have been developed to explore these difficulties (Happe, 1993).

The relationship between difficulties in acquiring and using language and the development of certain mental illnesses is currently receiving attention and suggests that language may be needed for the development of certain cognitive skills (Crow, 1998). However, it is difficult to be certain of the role of such a predisposing factor when the basis of an illness such as schizophrenia is not fully understood (Done, Leinonen, Crow et al., 1998).

This book has taken a particular perspective on semantic processing, which focuses on the semantic processing of language and what happens to semantic processing in clinical populations. This perspective has required us to largely ignore bigger questions of cognitive science, linguistics and philosophy in order to make sense of this area. Fodor (1998) reminds us that a better understanding of representations must be the aim. More importantly he states:

> The scientific goal . . . is therefore to understand what mental representations are and to make explicit the causal laws and processes that subsume them. Nothing about this has changed much, really, since Descartes.
>
> Fodor (1998: vii)

References

Bishop D (1997) Uncommon Understanding: Development and Disorders of Language Comprehension in Children. Hove: Psychology Press Ltd.

Boucher J (1998) SPD as a distinct diagnostic entity: logical considerations and directions for future research. International Journal of Language and Communication 33: 71–108.

Bryan K, Binder J, Funnell E, Ramsey V, Stevens S (1999) Language assessment in the elderly. Paper presented at the Clinical Neuropsychological Assessment Conference: October, London.

Byng S, Black M (1996) What makes a therapy? Some parameters of therapeutic intervention in aphasia. European Journal of Disorders of Communication 30: 303–16.

Byng S, Swinburn K, Pound C (1999) The Aphasia Therapy File. Hove: Psychology Press.

Caramazza A, Hillis AE, Rapp BC, Romani C (1990) The multiple semantics hypothesis: multiple confusions? Cognitive Neuropsychology 7: 161–89.

Cavanaugh JC (1983) Comprehension and retention of television programmes by 20–60 year olds. Journal of Gerontology 54: 1–22.

Cheshire J (1982) Linguistic variation and social function. In Romaine S, (Ed) Sociolinguistic Variation in Speech Communities. London: Edward Arnold. pp 153–75.

Constable A, Stackhouse J, Wells W (1997) Developmental word-finding difficulties and phonological processing: the case of the missing handcuffs. Journal of Applied Psycholinguistics 18: 507–36.

Couper-Kuhlen E, Selting M (1996) Towards an interactional perspective on prosody and a prosodic perspective on interaction. In Couper-Kuhlen E, Selting M, (Eds) Prosody in Conversation. Cambridge: CUP. pp 11–56.

Coupland N, Jaworski A, (1997) Sociolinguistics: A Reader and Coursebook. London: Macmillan Press.

Crow TJ (1998) Nuclear schizophrenic symptoms as a window on the relationship between thought and speech. British Journal of Psychiatry 173: 303–09.

Done DJ, Leinonen E, Crow TJ, Sacker A (1998) Linguistic performance in children who develop schizophrenia in adult life. British Journal of Psychiatry 172: 130–35.

Feil N (1992) Validation therapy with late-onset dementia populations. In Jones GMM, Meisen BML, (Eds) Care-giving in Dementia. London: Routledge. pp 199–218.

Fodor JA (1998) Concepts: Where Cognitive Science Went Wrong. Oxford: Oxford University Press.

Frith C (1997) Language and communication in schizophrenia. In France J, Muir N, (Eds) Communication and the Mentally Ill Patient. London: Jessica Kingsley.

Gardner-Chloros P (1997) Code-switching: language selection in three Strasbourg department stores. In Coupland N, Jaworski A, (Eds) Sociolinguistics: A Reader and Coursebook. London: Macmillan Press. pp 361–75.

Hamilton HE (1994) Conversations with an Alzheimer Patient. Cambridge: Cambridge University Press.

Happe FGE (1993) Communicative competence and theory of mind in autism: a test of relevance theory. Cognition 48: 101–19.

Holland AL (1990) Research methodology I: implications for speech-language pathology. ASHA Reports: 35–39.

Kemper S, Rash SR, Kynette D, Norman S (1990) Telling stories: the structure of adults' narratives. European Journal of Cognitive Psychology 2: 205–28.

Laver GD, Burke DM (1993) Why do semantic priming effects increase in old age? A meta–analysis. Psychology and Ageing 8: 34–43.

McGregor KK (1994) Use of phonological information in a word-finding treatment for children. Journal of Speech and Hearing Research 37: 1381–93.

Mogford-Bevan K, Sadler J (1992) Semantic pragmatic difficulties or semantic-pragmatic syndrome? Some explanations. In Mogford-Bevan K, Sadler J, (Eds) Child Language Disability, Vol. 2. Clevedon: Multilingual Matters.

Nickels LA, Best W (1996a) Therapy for naming deficits, Part 1: Principles, puzzles and progress. Aphasiology 10: 21–47.

Nickels LA, Best W (1996b) Therapy for naming deficits: Part 2: Specifics, surprises and suggestions. Aphasiology 10: 109–36.

Plaut DC, Shallice T (1993) Deep dyslexia: a case of connectionist neuropsychology. Cognitive Neuropsychology 10: 377–94.

Salthouse TA (1988) Effects of aging on verbal abilities: examination of the psychometric literature. In Light LL, Burke DM, (Eds) Language, Memory and Aging. New York: Cambridge University Press. pp 17–35.

Stackhouse J, Wells B (1997) Children's Speech and Literacy Difficulties – a Psycholinguistic Framework. London: Whurr.

Tager-Flusberg H (1991) Semantic processing in the free recall of autistic children: further evidence for a cognitive deficit. British Journal of Developmental Psychotherapy 9: 417–30.

Index